Cardiovascular Aspects of Marfan Syndrome

R. Hetzer, P. Gehle, J. Ennker
Editors

Cardiovascular Aspects of Marfan Syndrome

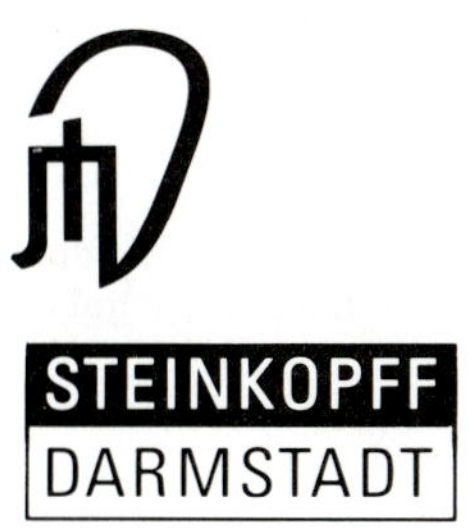

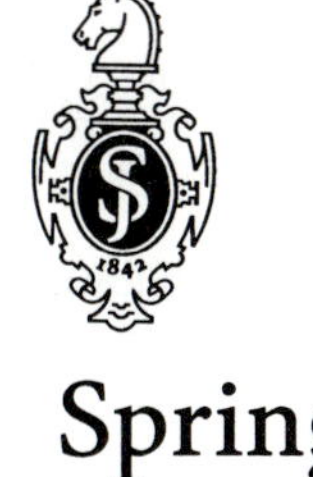

Springer

Prof. Dr. R. Hetzer
P. Gehle
PD Dr. J. Ennker
Deutsches Herzzentrum Berlin
Augustenburger Platz 1
13353 Berlin

Die Deutsche Bibliothek – CIP-Einheitsaufnahme

Cardiovascular aspects of Marfan syndrome / R. Hetzer ... (ed.). –
Darmstadt: Steinkopff, 1995
ISBN 3-7985-0959-X
NE: Hetzer, Roland [Hrsg.]

Medical Editor: Sabine Ibkendanz – English Editor: James C. Willis – Production: Heinz J. Schäfer

Printed in Germany

Typesetting, printing and bookbinding: VEBU Druck GmbH, Bad Schussenried
Printed on acid-free paper

Preface

The contributions in this volume were originally presented on October 16, 1993, at the Symposium on Cardiovascular Aspects of Marfan Syndrome in Berlin, FRG. The first part focuses on the underlying genetic defects and pathology in an attempt to clarify the cause and pathogenesis of the Marfan syndrome. The second part reviews the surgical techniques, and corresponding results, of eight experienced surgeons from Europe and the United States of America.

First described in 1896 by the Parisian pediatrician, Antoine Marfan, the Marfan syndrome remains enigmatic in several aspects. In 1931, Weve recognized the autosomally dominant inheritance of the disease, but nearly half a century passed until the responsible gene was found and could be localized on chromosome 15. A long succession of diligent researchers pioneered the path to our current understanding of the Marfan syndrome. In 1955, Victor McKusick created a nosology of heritable disorders of connective tissue concentrating on the Marfan syndrome (3). Although the syndrome's cardiovascular involvement was first described in 1942, most cases could only be diagnosed post mortem (5). It was first with the development of angiography, echocardiography, and sophisticated radiologic diagnostic methods, such as CT, spiral CT, and NMR scan, that early diagnosis and monitoring of the cardiovascular involvement of the Marfan syndrome became possible. Nevertheless, the primary factor in early diagnosis of the Marfan syndrome is the very act of considering if the symptoms presented indicate the presence of the syndrome. Following in the footsteps of McKusick, Reed Pyeritz has contributed greatly to the growing interest in the Marfan syndrome in the medical community. He has largely dedicated his professional life to basic and clinical research into the pathogenesis and clinical course of Marfan syndrome (4).

As Reed Pyeritz interestingly describes in chapter I, several teams of human geneticists who were intensively searching for a gene defect in the late 1980s agreed to coordinate their efforts such that each laboratory screened different chromosomes. Leena Peltonen's laboratory was able to localize the gene defect responsible for the Marfan syndrome on chromosome 15 in 1990.

Sally Allwork and Anton Becker, who extensively studied the cardiac pathology of Marfan patients, found very interesting specific features in Marfan aortas and coronary arteries. In particular, Becker's findings, which describe degenerative processes found in Marfan specimens and which are similar to those related to aging gave rise to lively discussion.

We also had the great honor of hearing a presentation by Hugh Bentall who developed a surgical technique for complete replacement of the ascending aorta and the aortic valve with a composite graft, which has remained the standard surgical procedure for over 25 years. It is well recognized that only since the introduction of this surgical technique was a clear step made towards the refinement of a relatively safe operation which can be accomplished with low mortality and few complications.

According to Paullin and James, first attempts at surgical treatment were made in the 1940s by Osler Abbott, who wrapped the ascending aorta in cellophane. It is known that the two patients he used this procedure on lived for at least 2 years, but were then lost during follow-up. One should also mention that Paullin, a long-time student of the problem of aortic dissection, died due to this condition. He diagnosed it with accuracy, insisted he could feel his aorta tearing, and correctly predicted that the rupture would take place into the left pleural cavity (2).

Operative procedures in the 1960s consisted primarily of aortic tubular replacements with or without separate valvular replacement, aortic wall wrapping, and/or valve resuspension (1). The main problem, potential dilation of sinu-aortal tissue, was not treated. Therefore, many of these early repair patients had to undergo reoperation for aortic root aneurysm.

More recently, Christian Cabrol's technique of linking the coronary ostia to the ascending graft with a separate "intercoronary" tube graft has found great acceptance since this procedure avoids tension on the coronary anastomoses and the potential of false aneurysm formation. Inberg's large series of Marfan patients who underwent surgery at his institution has become famous for indicating excellent results and meticulous follow-up. Joseph Coselli, colleague and successor of the late E. Stanley Crawford in Houston, presented his facility's vast clinical experience in aortic aneurysm surgery. In Germany, Hans Borst's equipe in Hannover has led in the field of thoracic aneurysm surgery for many years. His associate, Markus Heinemann, discussed these data. Francis Robiscek has contributed many original and sophisticated concepts and thoughts to all fields of cardiac and vascular surgery, including surgery of thoracic aneurysms and dissections.

Sir Magdi Yacoub has also introduced a great number of innovations to cardiac surgery. At our symposium, we were particularly indebted to him for his insightful comments about basic research and surgical decision-making and for sharing his immense experience in aortic valve-preserving procedures and in the use of homografts in Marfan patients, both of which have recently gained great interest worldwide. Finally, my colleague, Jürgen Ennker, presented the results of our work on a growing caseload of Marfan patients here in Berlin, including a few cases of possible Marfan-related pathology, such as cardiomyopathy and mitral valve dilatation and prolapse.

It is hoped that this book will serve as a timely synopsis of current knowledge about the pathogenesis, diagnosis and treatment of Marfan patients. We would like to thank each of the authors for undertaking the extra effort to contribute an article to this book. We are also indebted to Jonathan Davis, who transcribed the proceedings of the symposium, and to Sabine Ibkendanz and Jens Fabry of Steinkopff Verlag for their great patience in assembling and publishing this book. Our particular gratitude goes to Jeanine Fissenewert, my secretary, for her resoluteness and diplomacy in handling all of the extra work involved in arranging such an event, to Gerrit Jessen for his professionalism in organizing a smooth conference in a comfortable setting, and to the sponsors who through their generosity made the symposium feasible.

November 1994

Roland Hetzer
Petra Gehle

References

1. Berenson GS, Geer JC (1963) Heart disease in the Hurler and Marfan syndromes. Arch Int Med 111: 104–115, 1963 Jan
2. Burchell HB Aortic dissection (dissecting hematoma; dissecting aneurysm of the aorta). Circulation 12: 1068–79, 1955 Dec1
3. McKusick VA The cardiovascular aspects of Marfan's syndrome: a heritable disorder of connective tissue. Circulation 11: 321–42, 1955 Mar
4. Pyeritz RE The Marfan syndrome in: Connective tissue and its heritable disorders. Eds. Royce P, Steinmann B, New York, 1993, Wiley Liss, Inc., pp 437–468
5. Roberts WC, Honig HS The spectrum of cardiovascular disease in the Marfan syndrome: a clinico-morphologic study of 18 necropsy patients and comparison to 151 previously reported necropsy patients. Am Heart J 104(1): 115–35, 1982 Jul

Contents

Toward understanding cause and pathogenesis of Towards Marfan syndrome

R. E. Pyeritz

Department of Human Genetics, Allegheny-Singer Research Institute, Pittsburgh, Pennsylvania, USA

My task is to provide a foundation for the story Professor Peltonen and other speakers at this symposium will relate. My focus is the intellectual history that led to the recent discovery of the cause of the Marfan syndrome – an expedition that I always thought would lead to the pinnacle of any medical scientist's career, preferably mine. Having found the cause, however, we now realize that it is a false peak, just a foothill on the way to the summit. The presentations and discussion at this meeting will indicate how much further we all need to climb to achieve the goal of total understanding of this complex disorder.

I will not spend much time reviewing the clinical manifestations, although it is important to recognize Marfan syndrome as a pleiotropic disorder. All of the diverse clinical signs and symptoms derive from a single mutant gene [15, 16]. Professor Marfan, who I believe was the first physician designated a "Professor of Pediatrics" in the history of the world, recognized this important characteristic of pleiotropy within his own lifetime. By the 1930s, the skeletal involvement described by Marfan had been married to ocular problems and mitral valve problems, and there were strong indications that the phenotype was familial in a pattern consistent with mendelian dominant inheritance. What Professor Marfan did not appreciate about "his" syndrome was the cause of the premature mortality. Disease of the aortic root was not described until the 1940s, nearly 50 years after Marfan reported Gabrielle P., his first and perhaps only patient with this relatively common disorder.

It is appropriate that this symposium is being held in Berlin, because the diagnostic criteria for the Marfan syndrome were codified in this city in 1986, when a self-appointed group of experts gathered and promulgated their recommendations, which are widely used today [1]. These criteria are no different from any others that are based on bedside observation; they are far from perfect. The Marfan syndrome represents a clinical, or more precisely, phenotypic spectrum. At one end of the spectrum are patients about whom no one would debate; they have "classic" Marfan syndrome. Included among such patients are those called "neonatal Marfan syndrome", a designation I find counterproductive, because some physicians and scientists come away with the idea that these severely affected infants represent a different disorder. They do not. They simply were unfortunate to fall at the severe end of the phenotype. The other end of the Marfan spectrum is more accurately depicted as a continuum, where the phenotype gradually merges with the general population. All along this spectrum, various non-Marfan conditions overlap. Disorders such as autosomal dominant mitral valve prolapse syndrome (encompassed in its own spectrum we have termed the MASS phenotype [6]), various Ehlers-Danlos types, Stickler syndrome, familial aortic dissection, and others can, in individual cases, easily produce diagnostic dilemmas. The so-called Berlin criteria for the Marfan syndrome involve the family history in the decision matrix. If there is clearly an unequivocal case of Marfan syndrome in the family, then the person sitting in your consultation room requires less of a phenotype to be labeled as Marfan than would a patient with a negative or equivocal family history. The current criteria are summarized in the table.

In 1955, in an important paper on the cardiovascular manifestations of the Marfan syndrome, Victor McKusick [13] coined the term "heritable disorder of connective tissue". The next year, he published the first of four editions of a monograph entitled *Heritable Disorders of Connective Tissue* [14]. In the first and subsequent editions, the Marfan syndrome occupied the first chapter devoted to specific disorders, although osteogenesis imperfecta probably merited the position because it was interpreted as a systemic disorder of mesenchyme many years before. In the first edition, nine disorders were described in some detail. In the fifth edition, published last year as a multi-authored compendium, over 200 distinct disorders were listed as definitely or likely due to a defect in a single gene encoding a component of the extracellular matrix [2].

Finding the cause of the Marfan syndrome was long a "Holy Grail" of biochemists and geneticists. Forty years ago, it was clear that the search could proceed in two directions, exemplified by Fig. 1. This diagram represents a "pathogenetic tree", in which the phenotypic features are the leaves, the mechanisms by which the biochemical and cellular problems lead to the phenotype (that is, pathogenesis) are the branches and the trunk, and the actual genetic defect is the root. One could start by digging for the root, something like a frontal assault. Or, one could start by plucking leaves and working back through the foliage, along the brances, and eventually reach the root. Both approaches were tried, and a great deal of time, effort and resources led to considerable frustration. The literature is replete with false starts and epiphenomena, and I will not repeat a review of this history here [15]. Notice in the figure that the root is identified as a defect in elastic fibers. As we all now know, this is quite close to being an accurate description of the true cause, and it was suggested in 1955. But, for all his wisdom and insight, Professor McKusick could not be certain back then that his conjecture would prove correct, so he created multiple copies of this figure, identical except for the root. One version had a root identified as "collagen abnormality", while another had "mucopolysac-

Table 1. Diagnostic criteria for the Marfan syndrome [1].

If a first-degree relative is affected by the Marfan syndrome:
- The person under consideration must have:
  - Involvement of at least two systems;
  - At least one major manifestation (although this requirement is age-dependent and occasionally will depend on peculiarities of the family's phenotype).

If no first-degree relative is unequivocally affected by the Marfan syndrome:
- The proband must have:
  - Involvement of the skeleton;
  - Involvement of at least two other systems;
  - At least one major manifestation.

Suspected cases should have a plasma amino acid analysis in the absence of pyridoxine supplementation to document the absence of homocystinuria.

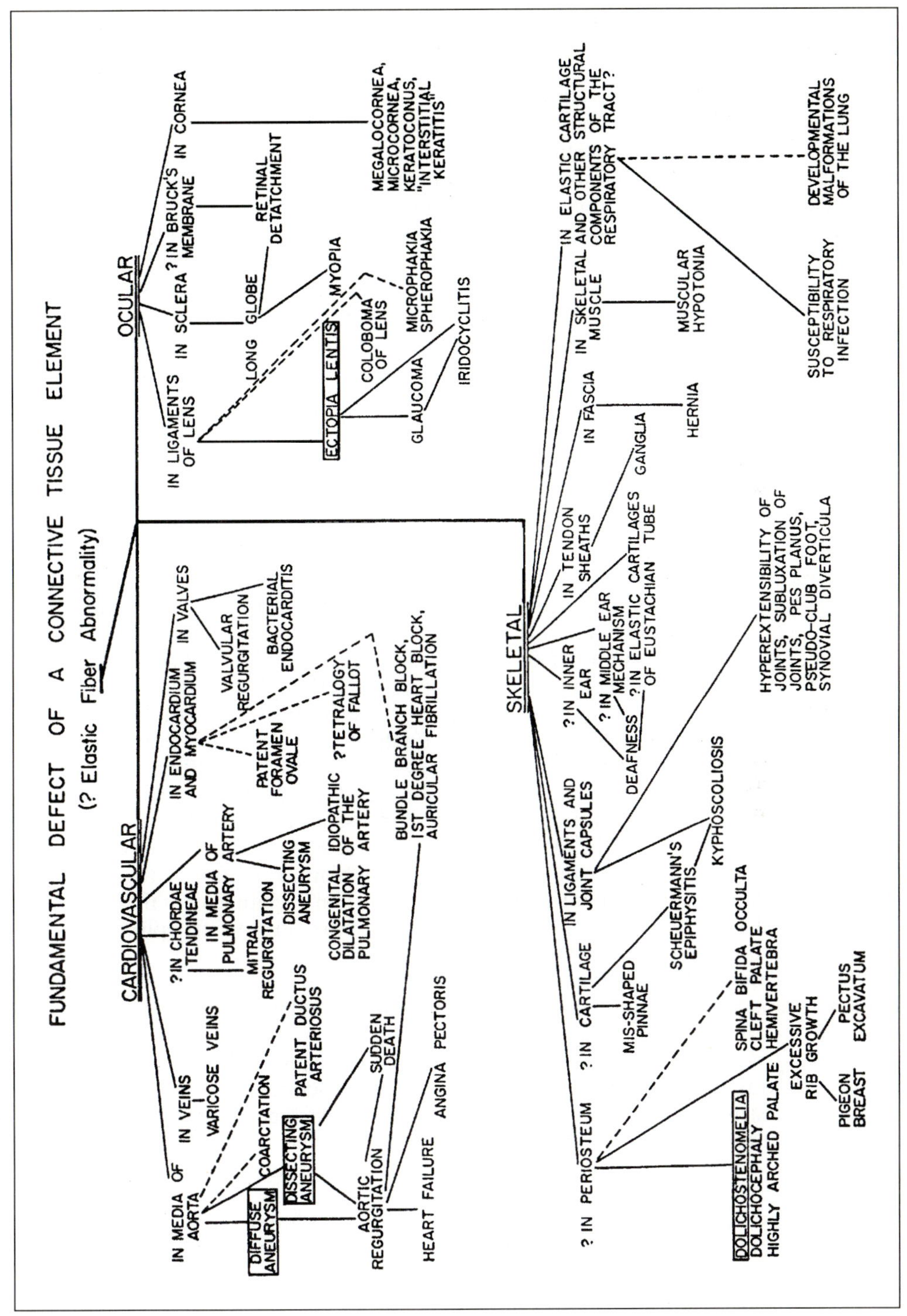

Fig. 1. Pathogenetic tree of the Marfan syndrome. From McKusick [13].

charide abnormality". To his credit, it was the "elastic fiber" version that was published, but I have the transparencies of the other versions to prove that he hedged his bets.

In the 1950s, it was clear that the aortic media is distinctly abnormal in the Marfan syndrome. The histopathology, termed "cystic medial necrosis" by Erdheim in 1930, proves to be a complete misnomer. There is neither necrosis nor cysts. The most striking feature is fragmentation and disarray of the elastic fibers. To be sure, the collagen fibers do not look normal either. What were called cysts are pools of excess accumulation of hyaluronate and proteoglycan. Professor Becker is the expert in this area, and if I say anything more, not only will I encroach on his presentation, but I will say something incorrect. Suffice it to say, the histopathology of the Marfan aorta provided plenty of opportunity over the years for biochemists to justify examining one or another of the components of the extracellular matrix, to no avail.

Another hallmark of the Marfan syndrome is ectopia lentis, with the lens typically displaced upward and the zonules stretched but intact [11]. McKusick, knowing of the evident importance of the zonules in keeping the lens in place, made the following prescient prediction in 1956 [14].

> "What the suspensory ligament of the lens has in common with the media of the aorta is obscure. If known, the basic defect of this syndrome might be understood".

It took more than 30 years to produce strong evidence of what that common link was, and another 4 years to prove it. For the remainder of this presentation, I will review the most important events that got us to where we are today.

In general, there are a number of intellectual approaches to finding the cause of a hereditary disorder. Biochemistry has been perhaps the most successful approach until relatively recently. The starting point is a tissue, in this case virtually any tissue because all contain an extracellular matrix. Each of the identifiable components of the extracellular matrix in turn is then scrutinized for something different compared to the same tissue from a person without the Marfan syndrome. Over the years, many biochemical "abnormalities" were found in tissues from Marfan patients, but as more was learned about the extracellular matrix in general, and other connective tissue disorders, it became clear that all of the biochemical components are highly integrated; altering one primarily results in secondary changes in many others. Thus, this classical approach to discovering cause was turning up epiphenomena, and was extremely frustrating for decades.

Another approach, possible only in the past 15 years, is to begin with a gene known to encode a component of the extracellular matrix. When I first became involved in connective tissue research, the extracellular matrix seemed so simple, even boring. There were a few fibrous elements – collagen and elastic fibers – and the amorphous ground substance. How many genes could possibly be involved? Perhaps a dozen? In fact, the extracellular matrix is extremely complex – there are at least 19 different collagen fibers, with each determined in all of their details by more than a dozen genes. Nonetheless, the genetic approach to heritable disorders of connective tissue has proven highly successful. In the most direct method, a gene known to encode one of the components of the extracellular matrix, or to encode an enzyme that modifies a component, is scrutinized for involvement in a specific disease. This can be done in one of two ways. The indirect method is linkage analysis, in which polymorphic markers in or near the gene of interest are examined in a family in which the disease is also present. If the same marker (which usually has nothing to do directly with the disease, but is simply a tag for which allele is being passed from parent to child) is present in all affected relatives, but not in unaffected relatives, then that gene is implicated. Obviously, the more relatives that can be typed, both genetically and phenotypically, the stronger the evidence, either for or against the association. This approach is termed the "candidate gene method".

Linkage analysis can only suggest a cause, not prove it. One always must go to the next step of finding a mutation in the gene (or its regulatory region) that is only present in people with the disease. Mutation-searching can be accomplished by a number of techniques, which Professor Peltonen will review.

What if all of the candidate genes available are scrutinized and none is the culprit? This happened in the Marfan syndrome by the mid-1980s. Markers throughout the human genome can be used in a "shotgun approach" to linkage analysis. These markers might (and today increasingly do) have no functional relationship to any known or even unknown gene. Rather, they serve as landmarks along individual chromosomes. If one marker is found to be linked to a disease, then by a process termed "positional cloning", the actual disease-causing gene is sought in the vicinity of the linked marker. This approach was used very successfully to locate and identify the genes for cystic fibrosis, Huntington disease, and the two forms of neurofibromatosis.

None of these methods was sufficient in and of itself to find the cause of the Marfan syndrome. This was the first mendelian disorder to be solved by a coalition of approaches, all conducted over a period of years, often in different parts of the world, but ultimately all pointing to the same notion. This was immensely reassuring to those of us conducting the research!

Recall the elastic fibers, so abnormal in the aortic media. They are composed of an amorphous core, consisting of highly cross-linked tropoelastin molecules, and a matrix of 10–12 nm diameter, long structures called extracellular microfibrils. Microfibrils are synthesized early in the genesis of the elastic fiber, and are the substructure for deposition and organization of tropoelastin. In addition, microfibrils exist throughout the body, often unassociated with elastin. Most importantly for this history, microfibrils are the zonules of the eye.

In 1986, Dr. Lynn Sakai and her collaborators at the Portland Shriners Hospital in Portland, Oregon, discovered and purified a very large glycoprotein, which she called fibrillin, that was found exclusively in the microfibrils [17]. Indeed, from the earliest work, it was suspected that fibrillin was the major structural protein of microfibrils. Purified monomers of fibrillin, of size 350 kD, spontaneously associated in vitro to form filamentous structures resembling microfibrils.

In collaboration with Dr. Sakai and the late Dr. David Hollister, I collaborated on studies that examined microfibrils in skin from patients with the Marfan syndroms, their unaffected relatives, and patients with other connective tissue disorders. We used an indirect immunofluorescent approach to histopathology that relied on monoclonal antibodies against fibrillin. There was strong evidence of both qualitative and quantitative abnormalities of microfibrils in patients with the Marfan syndrome [7].

At about the same time, Professor Peter Byers of the University of Washington in Seattle began examining the biochemistry of fibrillin produced by cultured skin fibroblasts. In collaboration with me, his fellow, Dr. Diana McGookey, showed that patients with the Marfan syndrome could be categorized into four classes. One group had difficulty synthesizing fibrillin. Another group synthesized it, but had difficulty secreting it from the cell. A third group made it, secreted it, but could not incorporated fibrillin in the extracellular matrix. Finally, there were a few patients who had no apparent abnormalities [12].

Finding abnormalities at the light-microscopic and biochemical level in skin was not surprising. One of the typical, pleiotropic clinical manifestations of the Marfan syndrome is striae atrophicae [15]. Microfibrils are abundant in skin and have been called various names by dermatologists over the years.

It was extremely reassuring to find that the abnormalities bred true in families, even at the level of the heterogeneity suggested by the different classes of patients based on biochemical analysis. These then were the crucial experiments that suggested fibrillin as role in the Marfan syndrome as worthy of pursuit as the "Holy Grail".

Simultaneously with this work, many laboratories, including ours at Johns Hopkins led by Dr. Clair Francomano, were attempting to localize the gene for the Marfan syndrome by linkage analysis. All candidate genes were excluded. Then, we and others turned to the shotgun approach. Out of frustration, we even talked with our competitors. The result was an international consortium of sorts, which pooled all linkage data and showed that nearly 90% of the human genome had been *excluded* as the location of the Marfan gene [3]. Few chromosomes or chromosomal regions had been ignored in this search. One that had been was chromosome 8. We directed our efforts there. Another was chromosome 15, and Professor Peltonen directed her efforts there. Hers was a much better choice. In looking at Finnish families with the Marfan syndrome, she and her collaborators found, in 1989, a linkage between the disorder and anonymous markers on the long arm of this chromosome, called 15q [8]. This was a tremendous accomplishment, and clearly focused all subsequent work at the molecular level.

We had been collaborating with Professor Bryan Hall at the University of Kentucky on evaluating a large family with over 100 people affected by the Marfan syndrome. Just before the first linkage was established, I took a young pediatric cardiologist, Dr. Harry Dietz, to visit this family in the hills of Appalachia. We conducted careful phenotyping (geneticists' language for clinical examination), always the first requirement for linkage analysis. We also obtained many blood samples for isolation of DNA. Once we knew the Grail was somewhere on 15q, Dr. Dietz, who had forsaken echocardiography for gel electrophoresis of DNA, and Dr. Francomano worked to refine the mapping of the Marfan syndrome locus [15]. A marker was found, D15S1, that showed no recombination with the Marfan syndrome in either the large Kentucky pedigree, or in any of the other families we were studying. (As it turns out, and totally unbeknownst to us in 1990, this marker is actually buried within the actual Marfan locus). This information localized the "Marfan gene" to a relatively narrow band of chromosome 15. While this band looks small on a diagram, there was enough DNA in the region of suspicion to encode hundreds of genes, so the search was clearly not over.

Neither we nor others had forgotten about fibrillin. Dr. Sakai and her group had succeeded in cloning the gene, and shared the sequence information with the Baltimore and Helsinki groups. We used the identification of a polymorphism within the fibrillin gene to map it to 15q [5], and Dr. Sakai also mapped the fibrillin gene to 15q using in situ hybridization [10]. Working independently, Professor Francisco Ramirez and his group in New York City also cloned the gene for this protein, and for another fibrillin-like protein. The first became known as FBN1 and the second, which they mapped to chromosome 5, was called FBN2 [9].

Thus, the stage was set to prove conclusively that mutations in the FBN1 gene cause the Marfan syndrome. This was accomplished by Dietz and colleagues when they found a single nucleotide change in the FBN1 gene that had the result of altering an arginine residue to a proline [4]. This is a change that could be predicted to be harmful, for at least three reasons. First, proline often alters the secondary structure of protein chains. Second, the region in which this mutation occurred was highly conserved; the sequence resembled epidermal growth factor, and the arginine residue was found in this position in similar EGF-like repeats present in proteins from very primitive organisms. Third, the arginine residue was postulated to be crucial for a hydroxylation reaction predicted to occur as a post-translational modification of fibrillin. Most telling, however, was the pedigree and population evidence. First, this specific mutation was not found in humans who did not have the Marfan syndrome; thus, it did not represent a common polymorphic nucleotide sequence variation. Second, neither of the patient's parents had the change. Neither of them had the Marfan syndrome; the patient was a sporadic case in the family, thought to be due to a new mutation in either the egg or the sperm that got together at her conception. The only firmer proof that might be desired is introducing this specific mutation into a transgenic mouse and producing the animal equivalent of the Marfan syndrome. This specific arginine -> proline mutation was found in the DNA of another patient; like the first, this girl had early onset of severe Marfan syndrome – what has sometimes been called the "neonatal Marfan syndrome". This has been touted as a separate phenotype, but is clearly just the severe end of the phenotypic spectrum of classic Marfan syndrome. This specific mutation has not been found in any other patient with the Marfan syndrome; in fact, thus far this is the only mutation in FBN1 that has occurred in two unrelated Marfan patients. As Professor Peltonen will relate, there are now (mid-1994) well over 4 dozen mutations in FBN1 known that cause Marfan syndrome, and only the first, termed R239P, has ever been found to have occurred independently more than once.

So, in mid-1991, the Grail had been discovered. Success was achived by a combination of approaches, although proof was by refined examination of the sequence of a candidate gene. But, as I intimated at the outset, discovering the cause was not the peak of the mountain. Understanding etiology enables rather limited clinical application, specifically in diagnosis. What all of us clinicians, (and especially our patients,) really desire are better ways of managing all of the pleiotropic manifestations. These methods will come about only by understanding how mutations in fibrillin are transformed into what we observe at the bedside. When we understand these processes – pathogenesis – we will be able to design targeted approaches to modulating the excessive growth of long bones, the laxity of ocular zonules, the weakness of the aortic media, and so on. This will keep us busy for quite a few years.

In closing, I would like to give proper credit to my collaborators and teachers, both at Johns Hopkins and elsewhere. Special thanks are due Dr. Lynn Sakai for sharing her discovery of fibrillin with us, Drs. Hal Dietz, Clair Francomano, and Garry Cutting for their tireless and expert molecular biology, and Prof. Victor McKusick, who in 1977, on my first day as a Senior Resident Physician on the Osler Medical Service at the Johns Hopkins Hospital, introduced me to a young man who just happened to have the Marfan syndrome. I became this boy's doctor, and the rest, as they say, is history.

References

1. Beighton P, de Paepe A, Danks D, Finidori G, Gedde-Dahl T, Goodman R, Hall JG, Hollister DW, Horton W, McKusick VA, Opitz JM, Pope FM, Pyeritz RE, Rimoin DL, Sillience D, Spranger JW, Thompson E, Tsipouras P, Viljoen D, Winship I, Young I (1988) International nosology of heritable disorders of connective tissue, Berlin, 1986. Am J Med Genet 29: 581–594
2. Beighton P (ed) (1993) McKusick's heritable disorders of connective tissue, 5th edition, C. V. Mosby Company, St. Louis
3. Blanton SH, Sarfarazi M, Eiberg H, de Groote J, Farndon PA, Kilpatrick MW, Child AH, Pope FM, Peltonen L, Francomano CA, Boileau C, Keston M, Tsipouras P (1990) An exclusion map of Marfan syndrome. J Med Genet 27: 73–77
4. Dietz HC, Cutting GR, Pyeritz RE, Maslen CL, Sakai LY, Corson GM, Puffenberger EG, Hamosh A, Nanthakumar EJ, Curristin SM, Stetten G, Meyers DA, Francomano CA (1991) Defects in the fibrillin gene cause the Marfan syndrome; linkage evidence and identification of a missense mutation. Nature 352: 337–339
5. Dietz HC, Pyeritz RE, Hall BD, Cadle RG, Hamosh A, Schwartz J, Meyers DA, Francomano CA (1991) The Marfan syndrome locus: Confirmation of assignment to chromosome 15 and identification of tightly linked markers at 15q15–q21.3. Genomics 9: 355–361
6. Glesby MJ, Pyeritz RE (1989) Association of mitral valve prolapse and systemic abnormalities of connective tissue: A phenotypic continuum. J Am Med Assoc 262: 523–528
7. Hollister DW, Godfrey M, Sakai LY, Pyeritz RE (1990) Immunohistologic abnormalities of the microfibrillar-fiber system in the Marfan syndrome. N Engl J Med 323: 152–159
8. Kainulainen K, Pulkkinen L, Savolainen A, Kaitila I, Peltonen L (1990) Location on chromosome 15 of the gene defect causing Marfan syndrome. N Engl J Med 323: 935–939
9. Lee B, Godfrey M, Vitale E, Hori H, Mattei M-G, Sarfarazi M, Tsipouras P, Ramirez F, Hollister DW (1991) Linkage of Marfan syndrome and a phenotypically related disorder to two different fibrillin genes. Nature 353: 330–334
10. Magenis RE, Maslen Cl, Smith L, Allen L, Sakai LY (1991) Localization of the fibrillin (FBN) gene to chromosome 15, band q21.1. Genomics 11: 346–351
11. Maumenee IH (1981) The eye in the Marfan syndrome. Trans Am Opthalmol Soc 79: 684–733
12. McGookey Milewicz D, Pyeritz RE, Crawford ES, Byers PH (1992) Marfan syndrome: Defective synthesis, secretion, and extracellular matrix formation of fibrillin by cultured dermal fibroblasts. J Clin Invest 89: 79–86
13. McKusick VA (1955) The cardiovascular aspects of Marfan's syndrome: A heritable disorder of connective tissue. Circulation 11: 321–342
14. McKusick VA (1956) Heritable Disorders of Connective Tissue. C. V. Mosby Company, St. Louis
15. Pyeritz RE (1993) The Marfan syndrome. In: Royce PM, Steinman B (eds). Connective tissue and its heritable disorders: Molecular, genetic and medical aspects. Wiley-Liss, New York, pp 437–468
16. Pyeritz RE (1989) Pleiotropy revisited: Molecular explanations of a classic concept. Am J Med Genet 34: 124–134
17. Sakai LY, Keene DR, Engvall E (1986) Fibrillin, a new 350-kD glycoprotein, is a component of extracellular microfibrils. J Cell Biol 103: 2499–2509

Author's Adress:
Prof. Reed E. Pyeritz
Department of Human Genetics
Allegheny-Singer Research Institute
320 E. North Avenue
Pittsburgh, PA 15212-4772 USA

Genetic basis of Marfan syndrome

L. Peltonen

National Public Health Institute, Helsinki, Finnland

Introduction

The informed clinician in the audience may realize, much better than a molecular biologist from Finland, how heterogenous the clinical phenotype of Marfan Syndrome is. It actually consists of a spectrum of clinical phenotypes. We all identify the classical Marfan Syndrome based on traditional criteria and like Dr. Pyeritz described, this disease was assigned to chromosome 15 some two years ago (1). But additionally, Marfan Syndrome consists of some other phenotypes; both very severe neonatal Marfan Syndrome, and a mild ectopia lentis, which I will discuss later, are also caused by a mutation in the same Marfan gene. Further, there is the mysterious "marfanoid" phenotype, of which we still know much too little to state anything definitive about the basic defect. Additionally, there are other very similar syndromes like contractural arachnodactyly which clearly is not caused by fibrillin on chromosome 15, but instead is most probably caused by mutations in the closely-related gene on chromosome 5 (9). Another related disease is familial annuloaortic ectasia for which only preliminary data exists on the molecular defect.

If we take a molecular biologist's view of Marfan genotype, we can state that, analogously to a spectrum of different phenotypes, there is a spectrum of different genotypes. At the DNA level, all possible mutation types have been identified in the Marfan patients on the fibrillin gene on chromosome 15 (3, 4, 5, 7). The only combining factor is this sizeable gene on chromosome 15, which is definitely defective at least in the majority of Marfan patients.

Our laboratory, like Dr. Pyeritz's laboratory, and several other laboratories around the world are extremely busy by screening and scanning through the fibrillin gene for different mutations in Marfan individuals. This is not just for the fun of identifying mutations, but rather to understand something about genotype/phenotype correlation in this mysterious disease, and to understand the functional significance of different parts of this gene and the corresponding polypeptide.

Fibrillin, the Marfan gene

The gene for fibrillin actually codes for an array of repeating structural domains and the white boxes shown in Fig. 1 represent 47 EGF-like motifs which are arrayed along the fibrillin polypeptide chain. The rigid structure of the polypeptide is, to a large extent, determined by these motifs, each containing six cys-residues and three disulfide bridges. The other structural motifs include 8-cysteine domains which carry high homology to TGF-β-binding protein. Thus, it is obvious that this protein is loaded with cysteines and this is one explanation why, most probably, the biochemical purification of this extracellular protein would have never solved the basic

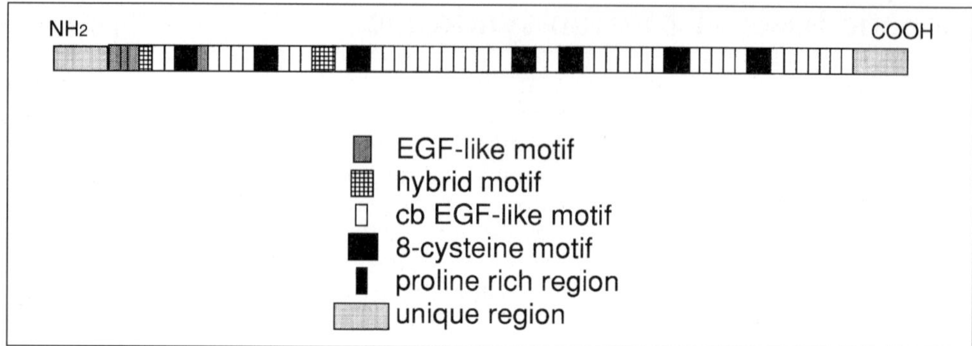

Fig. 1. Fibrillin.

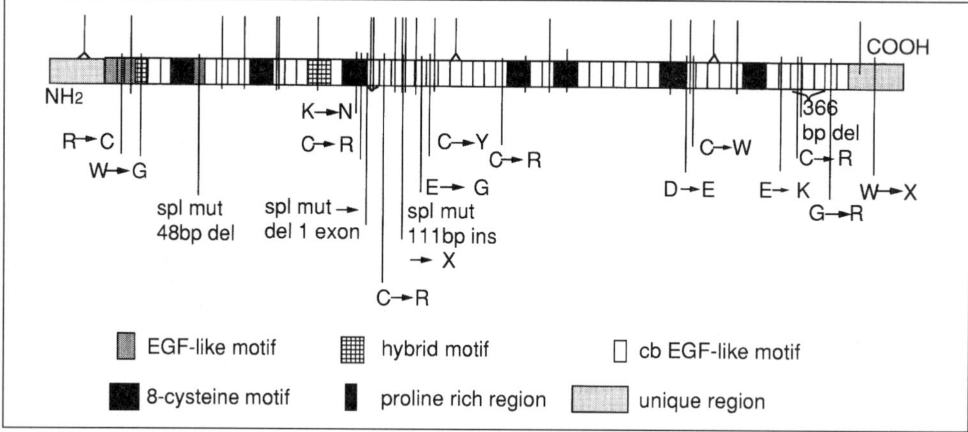

Fig. 2. Fibrillin mutations.

defect in the Marfan Syndrome. It is very difficult to purify from tissues or cell cultures since the molecules contain so many cysteines and form insoluble aggregates.

Figure 2 is somewhat complicated, but it should demonstrate all the so dar reported (nearly 40) mutations on the fibrillin gene in Marfan patients. As can be seen, the mutations occur at almost every position along this gene, and they represent a whole spectrum of mutation mechanisms. Based on these 40 mutations, the only thing we can positively state at this point is that the type of mutation or the mutated motif inside the fibrillin actually tells nothing about the genotype/phenotype relationship in this disease.

I would like to briefly illustrate how a molecular biologist proceeds in searching through the fibrillin gene to identify Marfan mutations. In Helsinki, we have a panel of cell lines from about 60 Marfan patients deriving from different European countries and also from some families in the USA. These patients represent both familial and non-familial cases. We typically grow fibroblast cultures from them, isolate genomic DNA, extract RNA, and then, (as detailed in Dr. Pyeritz's contribution) we screen with different methods the coding region of about 10 kilobases of fibrillin to discover DNA changes. Additionally, of course, we have a control group panel of about 100 individuals, including those married into the Marfan families, for the purpose of excluding polymorphisms when identifying a nucleotide change.

Currently, our success rate is not outstanding and neither is that of the other laboratories. Among these 60 individuals we have identified 20 different mutations. That is, we can identify one out of every three, and we hope to soon have a better yield by automated sequencing of the whole coding region. When one finds a mutation in the large gene, it is not a straight-forward task to establish that this nucleotide change actually causes the disease. First, one hase to confirm the finding in the genomic DNA, then, one has to screen other Marfan patients and also several controls in order to be sure that the finding really represents the mutation, and additionally, of course, one has to establish consegregation in the family, or, if it is a sporadic case, to demonstrate the absence of the mutation in the parents cell lines.

Deletions of the fibrillin gene

One specific group of fibrillin mutations produces shortened fibrillin polypeptide. There are several reasons why we have analyzed these mutations in detail. First, they are easy to identify. Since Marfan syndrome is a dominant disease, the disturbing fact is that, in most of the patients, the product of the healthy allele will also be present in their cells and tissues. Therefore one cannot simply go ahead and biochemically analyze fibrillin molecules in the patients fibroblasts, because half of the polypeptides will be normal and it is extremely difficult to identify normal from abnormal when there is just one amino acid difference. Whereas, if the protein is deleted due to the mutation, it is easy to use biochemical tools to identify an abnormal product from a normal one. That is why we first study polypeptides resulting from the premature terminations or from the deletion of the fibrillin gene.

There are currently at least three premature termination mutations reported by Dr. Hal Dietz and by our group (5, 6), and the mutation I will shortly describe here is actually a point mutation resulting in early truncation of the fibrillin polypeptide very close to the carboxy-terminal end of the fibrillin. The subject patient is a very classical Marfan patient and symptoms from all the three major tissues are summarized here. We know that both alleles are equally transcribed, there seems to be no intracellular retention or delayed secretion of the defective, shortened fibrillin and secretion of truncated molecules into the medium occurs. But it seems that the processing of pro-fibrillin to fibrillin is disturbed in the patients and causes the delay in the extracellular incorporation of the defective polypeptide. We have also identified two deletions in Marfan patients – one occurring at the 3' end, removing three EGF-like domains close to the COOH-end of the fibrillin gene, and, in another patient, only one EGF-like domain is removed but this occurs in the middle part of the fibrillin polypeptide chain. The carboxy-terminal deletion is found in a British family, where again, the disease phenotype represents a highly classical one. The clinicians had problems to define if some family members really were affected by Marfan Syndrome or not. We could demonstrate deletion mutation in this family in all affected individuals and the absence of deletion in healthy individuals. In the case of one 8-year-old boy (III/4), although he was tall and skinny, he was

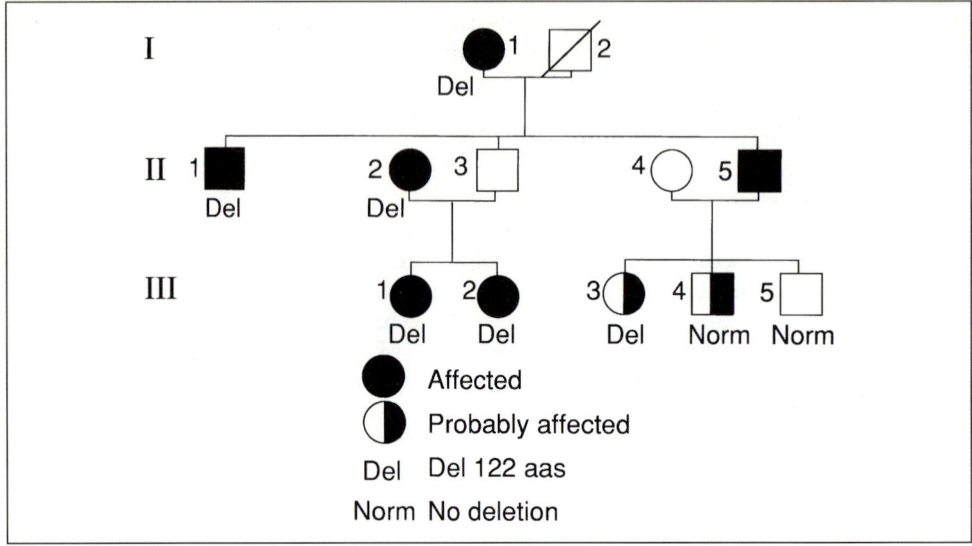

Fig 3.

shown definitely not to exhibit the Marfan mutation and he could be counselled to freely participate in all physical activities (Fig. 3). This is an example that in some families, we can already provide important information regarding individuals' health. The other deletion, occuring in the middle of the fibrillin polypeptide, I will return to, since this illustrates a very severe case of Marfan Syndrome.

Mutations in neonatal Marfan cases

Next I would like to shortly cover three severe neonatal Marfan cases which we have studied in collaboration with Dr. Beat Steinmann and Dr. Michael Raghunath from Zürich. These three patients represented very typical lethal cases of Marfan syndrome. Of the three mutations, one is the deletion of one EGF-domain, the two others represent different point mutations in the polypeptide chain. The only unifying feature besides the resulting phenotype is that they occur very close to each other in the fibrillin polypeptide chain. They occur at the beginning of the longest stretch of 12 repetitious EGF motifs. There are 12 EGF motifs following the 8 cysteine hybrid motif only once in the fibrillin polypeptide chain and it seems that when the mutation occurs in this region it somehow causes a very severely affected phenotype. Dr. Diana Milewicz (8) has studied an additional neonatal Marfan mutation which also occurs in this region, and we recall that the very first mutation which Dr. Hal Dietz (4) described is also located close to this region, thus further supporting the idea that this region is somehow of highest importance for the microfibril formation since different mutations at the DNA level actually produce strikingly similar, very severe Marfan phenotype.

What could be the explanation for this key region in the fibrillin molecule? There is actually an analogy existing in other systems, and what I mean by analogy is that in Drosophila there are similar EGF repeat motifs found in a specific locus

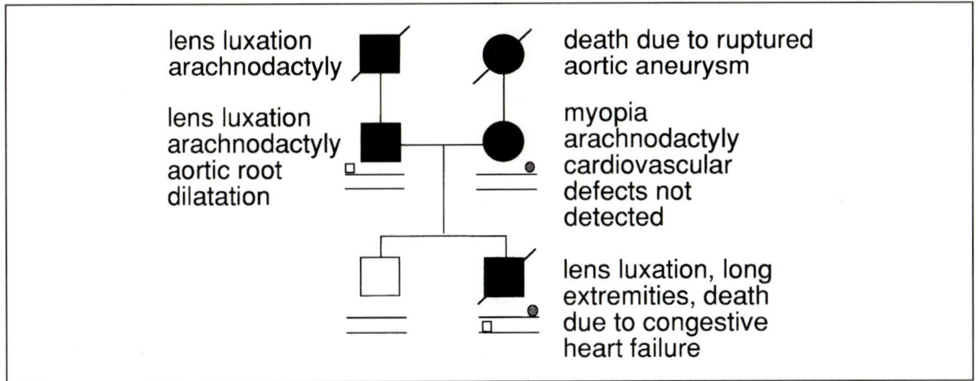

Fig. 4. Compound heterozygote.

whose function has been easily determined. Careful work from several laboratories (9) demonstrates that there is a clear differentiation of function in different EGF motifs based on their position in the polypeptide chain. Analogously, perhaps this particular position in the fibrillin polypeptide chain is somehow very important for the formation and/or stability of microfibrils.

With the next Marfan case I would like to remind you that all the severe affected Marfan individuals do not show mutations in this specific region of the gene. We have one severe Marfan patient whose parents were both rather mildly affected Marfan individuals. He actually turned out to be a compound heterozygote for two different mutations – the father carried a tryptophane to glycine mutation in the region coding for the amino terminal end of the polypeptide chain, and the mother carried a glycine to arginine mutation close to the COOH-end of the polypeptide chain. We could demonstrates that, the baby had inherited both and had a lethal form of the disease (Fig. 4).

Ectopia lentis and fibrillin gene

In addition to Marfan syndrome, also the phenotype dominatd by ectopia lentis is caused by mutations in the fibrillin gene. Figure 5 depicts a dominant ectopia lentis family which also has some skeletal symptoms; some individuals actually have only myopia and skeletal symptoms, and not dramatic ectopia lentis. The phenotype of the family thus closely resembles the first ectopia lentis family described in 1943 (10). Here we found a point mutation, changing lysine to arginine at a position very close to the COOH-end in the fibrillin polypeptide. The mutation G/A could always be found in the affected individuals and in the case of this family the mutation causes a disease which never progresses to the cardiovascular disease (11). There has not been a single clinical sign of cardiovascular involvement in four generations (Fig. 5). Thus it seems that the ectopia lentis mutation, i.e., the lysine to arginine mutation, results in marfanoid phenotype with no cardiovascular involvement. Why is this? We do not yet know the answer. In the immediate vicinity of this mutation on the fibrillin polypeptide there are mutations which result in classical Marfan phenotype. So here the explanation based on the position of the

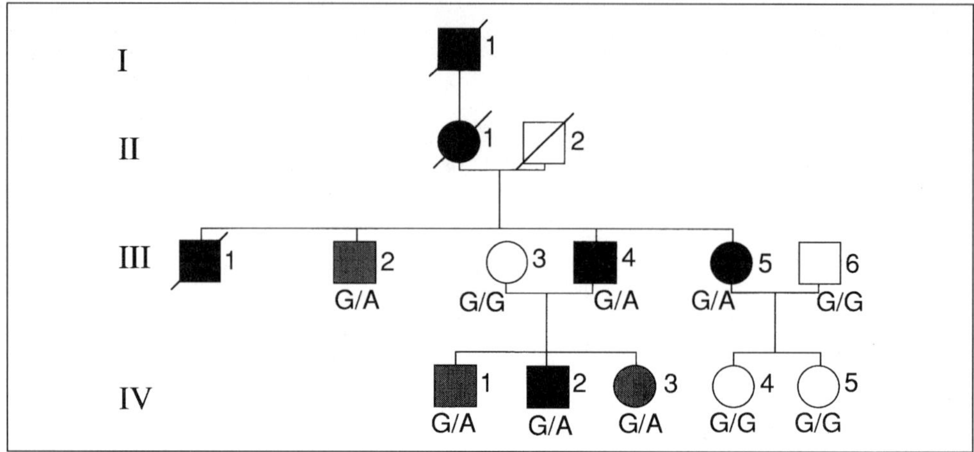

Fig. 5. Ectopia lentis-family.

mutation does not seem to hold. If the character of the mutation – this is the first lysine mutation in the EGF-repeat – is of significance, remains to be confirmed.

Genotype-phenotype correlation

What can we at this stage state about genotype/phenotype correlation based on the data from several groups around the world studying Marfan mutations? I believe most scientists in the field would state that there are no rules yet for this relationship, and although we can identify a mutation in an individual, we still cannot give that individual's prognosis or predict his or her symptoms. Some preliminary rules, however, might have emerged and I would like to suggest that mutations striking in the specific region in the beginning of the longest stretch of EGF repeats, could perhaps result in mutated polypeptides which become incorporated into the extracellular matrix and totally disrupt the microfibrils, resulting in exeptionally severe neonatal Marfan syndrome (12).

As Dr. Pyeritz has already pointed out, although we know the mutated gene behind Marfan syndrome and have a relatively well-defined disease, the consequences of Marfan mutations are not so evident and are rather enigmatic. We still have a lot of work to do and numerous demanding molecular techniques have to be applied before we can understand the genotype/phenotype relationship in this disease.

DNA diagnostics of Marfan syndrome

I will close with a few comments concerning DNA diagnostics of Marfan syndrome. If the patient represents a familial case and there are at least two individuals having Marfan syndrome in the family, we can provide a reliable DNA-diagnosis based on the use of intragenic polymorphisms (13). If the patient is the first case in the family, in only about one-third of the cases can we currently identify the mutation, and the remainder of the cases still remains without specific DNA diagnosis. With current sequencing technology, identification of unknown mutations is still a demanding and expensive effort. Consequently, only a limited number of patients have so far obtained immediate benefit from our molecular remove studies. However, in future these studies will without doubt help us to dissect the molecular pathogenesis of this multifacial disease called Marfan syndrome.

Acknowledgment

There is a long list of clinicians who, throughout the years, have actively collaborated with us; Here I would especially like to stress the role of the young medical student, Kati Kainulainen, who came to carry on a short scientific project in our laboratory and was able to identify the location of the Marfan gene. Also, the role of Dr. Lynn Sakai in identifying and cloning the fibrillin gene has been essential for our work. Our studies have been supported by the Academy of Finland.

References

1. Kainulainen K et al. (1990) Location on chromosome 15 of the gene defect causing Marfan syndrome. New Engl. J. Med. 323, 935–939
2. Tsipouras P et al. (1992) The international Marfan syndrome collaborative study: Genetic linkage of the Marfan syndrome, ectopia lentis, and congenital contractural arachnodactyly to the fibrillin genes on chromosomes 15 and 5. New Engl. J. Med. 326, 905–909
3. Lee B et al. (1991) Linkage of Marfan syndrome and a phenotypically related disorder to two different fibrillin genes. Nature 352, 330–334
4. Dietz, HC et al. (1991) Marfan syndrome caused by a recurrent de novo missense mutation in the fibrillin gene. Nature 352, 337–339
5. Kainulainen K et al. (1992) Two mutations in Marfan syndrome resulting in truncated fibrillin polypeptides. Proc. Natn. Acad. Sci. 89, 5917–5921
6. Dietz HC et al. (1993) Significance for mutant transcript level and EGF-like domain calcium binding in the pathogenesis of Marfan syndrome. Genomics 17, 468–475
7. Dietz HC et al. (1992) Marfan phenotype variability in a family segregating a missense mutation in the epidermal growth factor-like motif of the fibrillin gene. J. Clin. Invest. 89, 1674–1680
8. Milewicz DM, Dubiv M Severe neonatal Marfan syndrome resulting from a de neve three base pair insertion into the fibrillin gene on chromosome 15. Am. J. Hum. Genet., in press
9. Kelly MR et al. (1987) Mutations altering the structure of epidermal growth factor-like coding sequences at the drosophila Nutch locus. Cell 51, 539–548
10. Falls HF Cotterman CW (1943) Genetic studies on ectopia lentis: A pedigree of simple ectopia of the lens. Arch. Ophthal. 30, 610–620
11. Lönnqvist L et al. (1994) A novel mutation of the fibrillin gene causing ectopia lentis. Genomics 19, 573–576
12. Kainulainen K et al. (1994) Mutations in the fibrillin gene responsible for dominant ectopia lentis and neonatal Marfan syndrome. Nat. Genet. 6, 64–69
13. Rantamäki T et al. (1994) DNA Diagnostics of the Marfan syndrome: Application of amplifiable polymorphic markers. Eur. J. Hum. Genet. 2, 66–75

Author's address:
Leena Peltonen, MD, Ph. D.
National Public Health Institute
Mannerheimintie 166
00300 Helsinki
Finland

Cardiovascular disease in Marfan patients in infancy and childhood

Sally P. Allwork, Vivienne M. Miall-Allen, Richard K. Wyse, James F. N. Taylor

Cardiothoracic Unit, The Hospital for Sick Children London, England

The case of Gabrielle P, aged 5½ months, gave no indication that there was any cardiovascular involvement; and there is now some doubt that Marfan patient actually had the eponymous disease [6, 8].

The first case with cardiovascular disease was also the first description of Marfan syndrome in infancy. The German paediatrician Salle described a patient with failure to thrive and progressive dyspnoea who died at 2½ months of age. Autopsy demonstrated cardiomegaly and thickened mitral and tricuspid valves, both with redundant leaflet tissue [12].

The infant or child who presents with cardiovascular manifestations of Marfan syndrome (rather than actively seeking signs of the disease), has a worse prognosis than the patient presenting in adolescence.

Presentation of cardiovascular disease itself (rather than looking for the manifestations) implies a more severe affectation. Other children present either because they are from known Marfan families, or they have ocular manifestations, or have kyphoscoliosis or pectus excavatum, or because they are remarkably tall for their age, or because they seem to have stopped growing. By contrast, in infancy and young childhood the usual manifestation is cardiac failure, often with mitral valve dysfunction; typically annual dilatation, and long, malformed leaflets with mitral valve prolapse, often severe. Average age at death for patients presenting in infancy is 16.3 months as opposed to 33.5 years for those diagnosed in adolescence [8]. Death in the infant group results from congestive heart failure secondary to mitral valve regurgitation with or without aortic valve regurgitation, while in older patients the commonest cause of death is aortic dissection and/or rupture.

In infants tricuspid regurgitation occurs in 67% of cases and pulmonary valve regurgitation in 22%. Both of these are uncommon in older patients [5].

Pulmonary abnormalities such as bullae and emphysema add to the mortality in this age group and may be exacerbated by pectus excavatum or pectus carinatum. Joint deformities, notably laxity, but sometimes contracture, are also associated with the most profound cardiovascular changes. Ectopia lentis is also often noted.

Congenital malformations of the heart

In both Marfan syndrome and in congenital contractual arachnodactyly, congenital cardiac malformations co-exist with some frequency, probably exceeding the generally accepted norm of 8/1000 live births [5]. The anomalies range from relatively minor interatrial communications (Fig. 1) to Fallot's tetralogy (Fig. 2a, b).

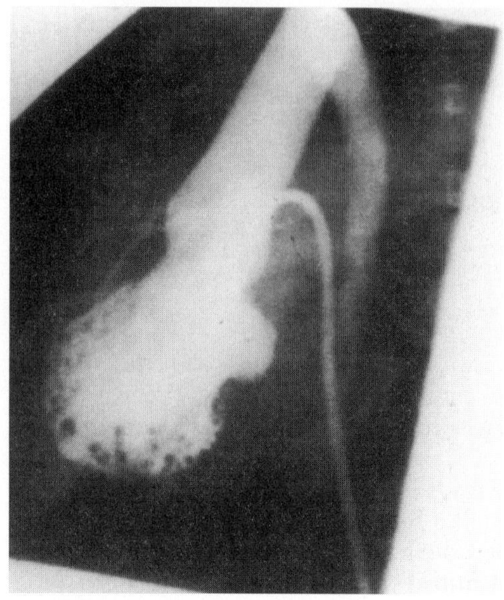

Fig. 1. Left ventricular angiocardiogram in a 5-year-old with Marfan's syndrome. The route of the catheter demonstrated an interatrial communication and mild mitral valve regurgitation.

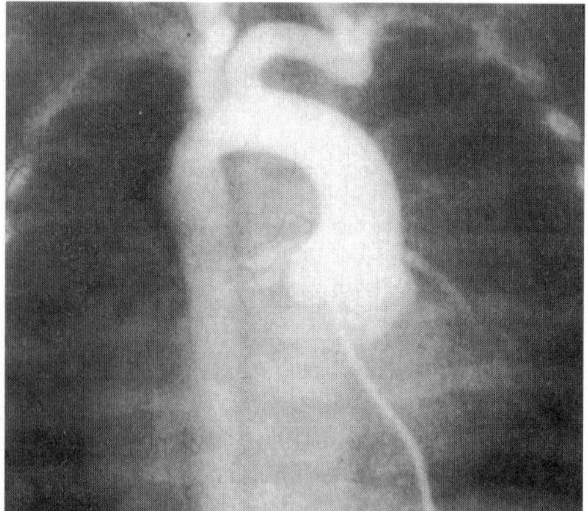

Fig. 2a. Antegrade antogram in a 2-year-old with Fallot's tetralogy.

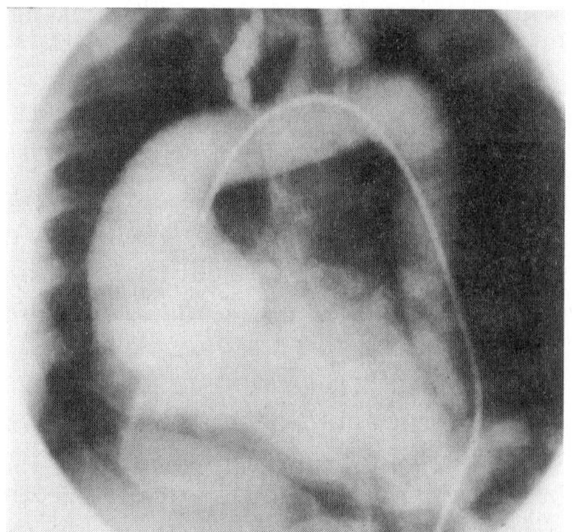

Fig. 2b. The same patient aged, after repair of the Fallot's tetralogy. The aortic root and ascending aorta are markedly dilated and there is kyphoscoliosis. Her parents had observed that growth had apparently ceased.

Aortic root involvement is the major cause of mortlity in older Marfan patients (adolescents and adults), but rare in babies and young children. In adults, "Type A" dissection (ascending aorta) is the leading cause of death, with "Type B" accounting for less than 20% of fatal dissection. (This contrasts with the well recognised pattern of aortic dissection and/or rupture due to other causes, where type A dissection is the least common) Although dissection is uncommon in the younger patients, aortic valve regurgitation is often present [5] and is progressive. However, the largest aortas are not necessarily those most likely to dissect, although irrespective of underlying pathology, any aorta whose diameter is 6 cm or more is likely to be unstable.

The anatomy of the aortic root

The aortic outflow tract is mainly fibrous. It comprises the aortic valve, the membranous part of the ventricular septum, the area of aortomitral fibrous continuity and the infundibular septal muscular portion which supports the right aortic leaflet and aortic sinus (1).

The elastic media of the aorta terminates at the aortic bar, just above the aortic sinus, so that the aortic "annulus" is generally devoid of elastic. (It should be noted that although for surgical purposes there is a readily recognisable aortic ring, i.e. the junction between the ventricle with muscle and the line of "attachments" of the aortic sinuses, in anatomical terms it does not really exist.)

This morphology is established early in fetal life. Histologically the adult arrangement of the aorta, (intima, 29 rows of elastin and smooth muscle cells and collagen forming the media, together with a vascular adventitia) are present from birth (Fig. 3). During the perinatal week there is a rapid accumulation of both elastin and collagen especially in the distal (including abdominal) aorta which is not related to the flow changes that occur at birth [3].

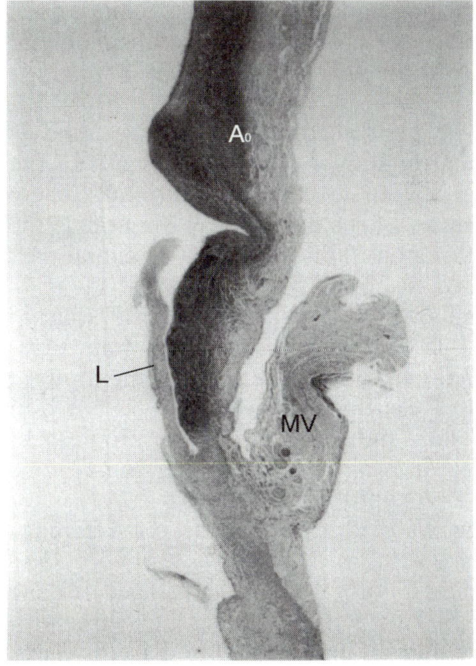

Fig. 3. Saggital section through the aortic root in a 24-week fetus. The aorta is structurally similar to that of an adult. Note that the elastic tissue does not extend to the "hinge" of the aortic valve leaflet. Ao = Aorta, L = aortic valve leaflet, MV = mitral valve – (Elastic Van Gieson, original magnification X 4).

Although they do not extend into the aortic sinus, elastic fibres, which are composed of elastin deposited on microfibrils, are relatively more abundant in the proximal ascending aorta than in any other artery, so that it is reasonable to assume that this morphology, together with the repetitive expansile stresses of left ventricular ejection, may be responsible for the early aortic dilatation that characterises the cardiovascular aspect of Marfan syndrome [11].

Although the coronary arteries are the only branches of the ascending aorta, they, unlike the aorta, continue to elaborate as young life advances. In fetuses and also in infants the usual arrangement of intima, media and adventitia is established, but the proportions vary. Up to a year of age the media in the most proximal coronary arteries is only 5–6 rows of smooth muscle cells and elastic fibres thick, and does not assume the adult pattern (up to 20 rows) until later in childhood (2). The author has often observed that patients with Marfan syndrome have coronary arteries that are relatively small in diameter. In normal adult men the proximal part of the anterior descending branch of the left coronary artery usually exceeds 6 mm diameter, that of normal women being up to 6 or 7 mm, whereas in Marfan syndrome, 4–5 mm is the usual finding in both sexes.

Aortic root enlargement in infancy and childhood

Although aortic valve regurgitation is often present in infancy, enlargement of the aortic root occurs in later childhood and particularly in adolescence. Monitoring of aortic root dimension is feasible with echocardiography but correlation of the results with angiocardiography is poor, as the two modalities do not recognise the same parameter. Furthermore, not only is there no accord about which phase of the cardiac cycle to choose for measurement, but standardisations for comparison are difficult to obtain in children: body surface area, for example, is unsuitable in Marfan syndrome, as height may greatly exceed the normal for age, while weight is far below it.

In order to overcome these difficulties we performed a retrospective analysis of video recordings of cross-sectional echocardiography of the aortic root in the parasternal long axis view. A measurement was made at four points (10). These were the aortic "annulus" (region 1), the sinuses of the aortic valve, (region 2) the sinutubular junction (i.e. at the aortic base) (region 3) and the most proximal part of the ascending aorta (region 4) (Fig. 4).

Images were obtained using an ATL Ultramark 8 or 9 ultrasound system utilising a 5 or 3.5 mHz mechanical sector scanhead. In each case the chosen frame corresponded to the optimal parasternal long axis view, and the measurements were made at the enddiastolic point of the cardiac cycle. Body surface area was noted in each case. Reference range was 95% confidence limit relating with the progression line for dimension against surface area, based on measurements of the four regions made in 327 normal children.

The dimensions in the Marfan patients were plotted against the reference ranges.

Study population. Echocardiograms from 327 normal individuals, aged from 1 week to 30 years were reviewed and compared with those from 26 patients with Marfan syndrome. The patients, from 20 families, were aged from 5 to 20 years,

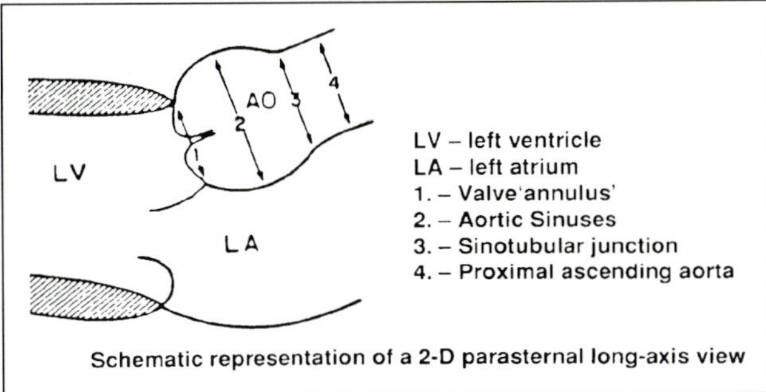

Fig. 4. Diagram to indicate the two-dimensional parasternal long axis echocardiographic image and the four points at which measurements were made.

and each had an echocardiogram on every visit to the hospital. The visits ranged in number from 1–11, the average being 3–4 per patient.

Results. The site of aortic dilatation in the Marfan patients was region 2 (the aortic sinus). This dilatation gave the characteristic "flask-shaped" aortic root. The aortic annulus, the sinutubular junction and the proximal ascending aortic dimensions all varied parallel to the reference range, but within the mean and the 95 % confidence limits (Figs. 5–8), but region 2 (the sinuses) was always disproportionally large, even in young children.

As childhood advances, dilatation of the aorta in Marfan patients is less uniform, so that it is possible that two divergent patterns emerge in patients aged 13 years and above (BSA 1.4m2). One group showed that all measurements continued to grow parallel to the reference range, while in the other all measurements accelerated rapidly away. In both groups, the enlargement was greatest in region 2 (Fig. 9). Aortic valve dysfunction may occur as adult dimension is reached, but this was not found to be related directly to the individual dimensions.

Discussion

None of the patients in this series had an aortic root of 5 cm or more in diameter, and to date, none has developed aortic dissection. It seems likely that once the aorta has begun to dilate, stresses on the surrounding structures, especially the ascending aorta, will bc abnormal, and this is likely to lead to even further enlargement.

Some patients appear to show a greater tendency to accelerated dilatation than others, but a greater number of patients followed from childhood to adolescence will be required for confirmation. This study does not suggest a direct correlation between aortic root dimensions and dissection of any part of the aorta.

In infants, the burden of cardiac manifestation of Marfan syndrome is borne by the mitral valve. It is not known at present whether this represents a different expression of the fibrillin gene, or simply a different structural abnormality of fibrillin. The youngest patients presenting in cardiac failure have the worst prognosis, particularly if there is a positive family history. There is no evidence that the infants

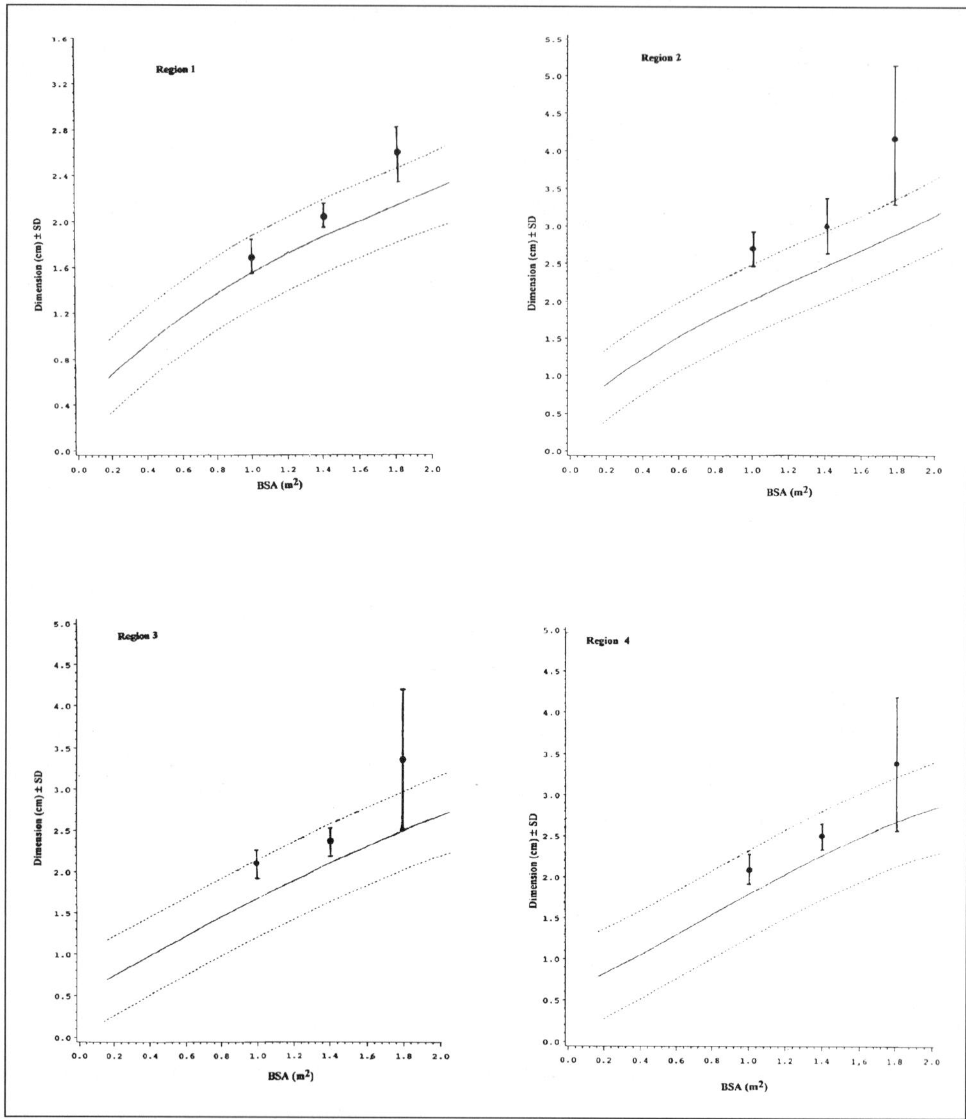

Fig. 5. The results of the measurements in all four regions.

have a different gene abnormality (e.g. on chromosome 5 rather than 15), but there may be a different fibrillin abnormality. The prognosis is also adversely affected if aortic root dimension exceeds 5 cm [13]. The long-term results of both medical and surgical therapy are disappointing in the youngest patients [13], so that it seems likely that effective drug therapy would be aimed towards enhancing the aortic wall structure to resist the stresses in the aortic wall during growth, especially during the pubertal "growth spurt". The therapy should modify response during exercise in the growth period as well as at rest.

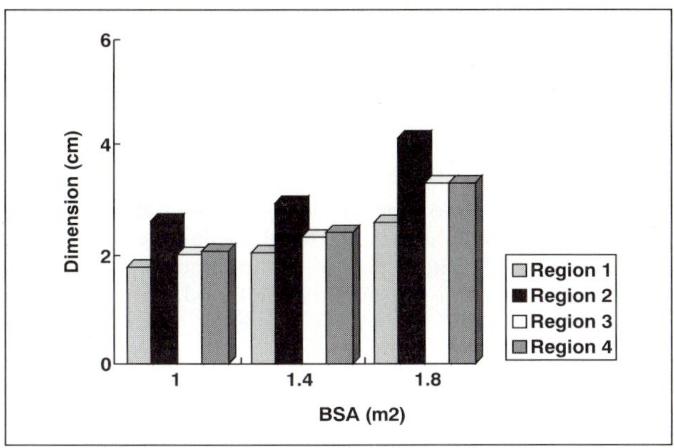

Fig. 6. Summary of the results showing the rapid acceleration away from the confidence limits in some patients as adult dimension is reached.

Conclusions

The cardiovascular aspects of Marfan syndrome in infancy and very early childhood carry a high mortality and are aggravated by both pulmonary and skeletal abnormalities. Aortic dilatation in older children begins in the aortic sinuses before puberty and in some patients rapidly accelerates thereafter, while in others dilatation proceeds more slowly. The onset of dilatation occurs at the junction of "elastic" and inelastic portions of the aortic root.

References

1. Allwork SP (1986) The anatomical basis of Infection of the Aortic Root. Thoracic Cardiovasc Surg. 34: 143–148
2. Allwork SP (In Press) the Anatomy of the Coronary Arteries In: The Atlas of Coronary Heart Disease. D G Julian Ed. Science Press; London
3. Bendeck MP, Langville BL (1991) Rapid Accumulation of Elastin and Collagen in the Aortas of Sheep in the immediate Postnatal Period Circ Res 69: 1165–1169
4. Dietz HL, Cutting GR, Pyeritz RE; Maslen CL, Sakai LY, Puffenberger EG, Hamosh A, Nanthakumar J, Curristin SM, Stetten G, Meyers DA & Francomano CA (1991) Marfan syndrome caused by a recurrent de novo missense mutation in the fibrillin gene. Nature 352: 337–339
5. Geva T, Hegesh J, Frand M (1987) The clinical course and echocardiographic features of Marfan's syndrome in childhood. Am J Child 141: 1179–1182
6. Hecht F, Beals RK (1971) "New" syndrome of congenital contractual arachnodactyly originally described by Marfan in 1896. Paediatrics 49: 574–579
7. Lee B, Godrey M, Vitale E, Hisaeh Matte 1 M-G, Tsipouras P, 1991 (CCA) Ramiraz F, Hollister DW (1991) Linkage of Marfan syndrome and a phenotypically related disorder to two different fibrillin genes. Nature 352: 330–334
8. Marfan AB un cas de déformation congénitale des quatre membres, plus prononcée aux extrémetiés, charactérisée par l'allongement des os, avec un certain degré d'amincissiment. Bull Mem Soc MeD Hôp. (Paris) 13: 220–226

9. Maslen CL, Corson GM, Maddox BK, Glanville RW & Sakai LY (1991) Partial sequence of a candidate gene for the Marfan syndrome. Nature 352: 334–337
10. Miall-Allen VM, Taylor JFN, Rees PG, Allwork SP, Howarth SG (1991) Comparative aortic root measurement in controls and in children and adolescents with Marfan's syndrome. Brit Heart J. 66: 51 (Abstr)
11. Pyeritz RE (1993) Marfan Syndrome; Current and future Clinical and Genetic Management of Cardiovascular Manifestations. Sem Thorac Cardiovasc Surg 5: 11–16
12. Salle V (1912) Über einen Fall von angeborener abnormer Grobe der Extremitäten mit einen an Acromegalie erinnernden Symptomenkomplex. Jahrbuch der Kinderheilkunde 75: 540–550
13. Zahra KG, Hensley C, Glesby & Pyeritz RE (1989) The impact of medical and surgical therapy on the cardiovascular prognosis of the Marfan syndrome in early childhood. (Abstr) J Amer Coll Cardiol 13: 119A

Authors' address:
S. P. Allwork, M.D.
Cardiothoracic Unit
The Hospital for sick Children
Great Ormond Street
London WC1N 3JH

Cardiovascular pathology in Marfan syndrome – An overview

A. E. Becker

Department of Cardiovascular Pathology, University of Amsterdam, Academic Medical Center, Amsterdam, The Netherlands

Introduction

The clinical presentation of arachnodactyly, better known as Marfan syndrome, has been recognized for almost 100 years, but it is only relatively recent that McKusick (4) described the clinical presentation in detail and, moreover, identified the syndrome as an inherited connective tissue disease. Despite the heterogeneity in the phenotypic expression of the disease, Marfan syndrome was subsequently characterized as an autosomal dominant connective tissue disorder (5). Marfan syndrome occurs with an estimated preference of 1 : 10 000; the majority being familial, but approximately 15–30% of the patients are sporadic (5). The phenotypic features of Marfan syndrome vary, but include skeletal, ocular and cardiovascular manifestations. The skeletal symptoms of Marfan syndrome include increased height, disproportionally long limbs and digits and anterior chest deformities. The typical ocular findings include myopia and subluxation of the lenses. The most serious and often life-threatening manifestations of Marfan syndrome occur in the cardiovascular system. Aortic root dilation and aneurysm formation of the ascending aorta are the most prominent and aortic wall rupture, with or without aortic dissection, is a common cause of death.

This overview will concentrate on the cardiovascular pathology only.

Molecular genetics

The unravelling of the genetic background of Marfan syndrome was a significant task. Histopathologic studies had shown unequivocally that the supportive connective tissues were affected, but it remained unclear whether the primary fault was in the collagens, the elastin or in the extracellular matrix. The characterization in 1986 of fibrillin, a hitherto unknown extracellular matrix glyco-protein, by Sakai et al. (6) proved to be a major break-through. It soon appeared that a deficiency in the fibrillin immunofluorescence pattern, using monoclonal anti-bodies against the fibrillin polypeptide, was almost a constant finding in skin sections and fibroblast cultures of Marfan patients (1, 2). These findings, therefore, strongly suggested that a deficiency in fibrillin was intimately related to the genetic defect causing Marfan syndrome. Eventually, the group of Peltonen (3), using the linkage approach, succeeded in establishing a "Marfan locus" on chromosome 15. Since then, it has been shown that other mutations also may lead to the Marfan phenotype, all linked to genes coding for microfibrillar proteins (see L. Peltonen, this volume, page 9).

Table 1. The major pathologic conditions affecting the cardiovascular system in Marfan syndrome and their clinical consequences

Pathologic condition	Clinical consequences
Dilation of ascending aorta	Aortic dissection and/or rupture
Annulo-aortic ectasia aneurysms of sinus of valsalva	Aortic valve regurgitation*
Floppiness of aortic valve	Aortic valve regurgitation*
Floppines of mitral valve	Mitral valve regurgitation*
Dilation of mitral valve annulus	

* In some patients heart failure may ensue out of range with the degree of valve insufficiency.

Cardiovascular pathology

The cardiovascular sequelae of the fibrillin deficiency (see above) appear to relate directly to weakening of the supportive tissues. An overview of the major pathologic conditions affecting the cardiovascular system and their clinical consequences is provided in Table 1.

Aortic pathology

The aorta in patients with Marfan syndrome may present a variety of abnormalities, all of which share the feature of dilation. The ascending aorta may show severe fusiform dilation of the lumen with thinning of the aortic wall. Similarly, the aortic root may be affected, either as part of the dilated ascending aorta or in isolation. The latter condition is known also as annulo-aortic ectasia. Occasionally, patients may be encountered with annulo-aortic ectasia without any other phenotypic signs of Marfan syndrome. It remains as yet unsolved whether or not these cases should be considered as "formes frustes" of Marfan. There is evidence that degenerative connective tissue disease, related to "wear and tear" rather than a prime genetic defect, plays a role particularly in elderly patients (unpublished observations). Floppiness of the aortic valve has been reported to occur in patients with Marfan syndrome, although the histologic characteristics (see below) are often consistent with secondary changes induced by longstanding valve regurgitation rather than expressing a basic connective tissue defect.

The clinical consequences of the pathologic conditions of the aorta alluded to above are serious. Dilation of the aortic root may cause severe aortic valve insufficiency and, eventually, may cause progressive left heart failure. In some patients heart failure is rapidly progressive and much more severe than anticipated from the degree of valve insufficiency only. In this context the question has been raised, therefore, whether the basic defect in the coding for microfibrillar components of the connective tissues also may affect the integrity of the myocardial collagen meshwork. This remains as yet a matter of further investigations.

The major catastrophe that can occur is that of aortic wall rupture, with or without aortic dissection (Fig. 1). Since the pathology affects the ascending aorta,

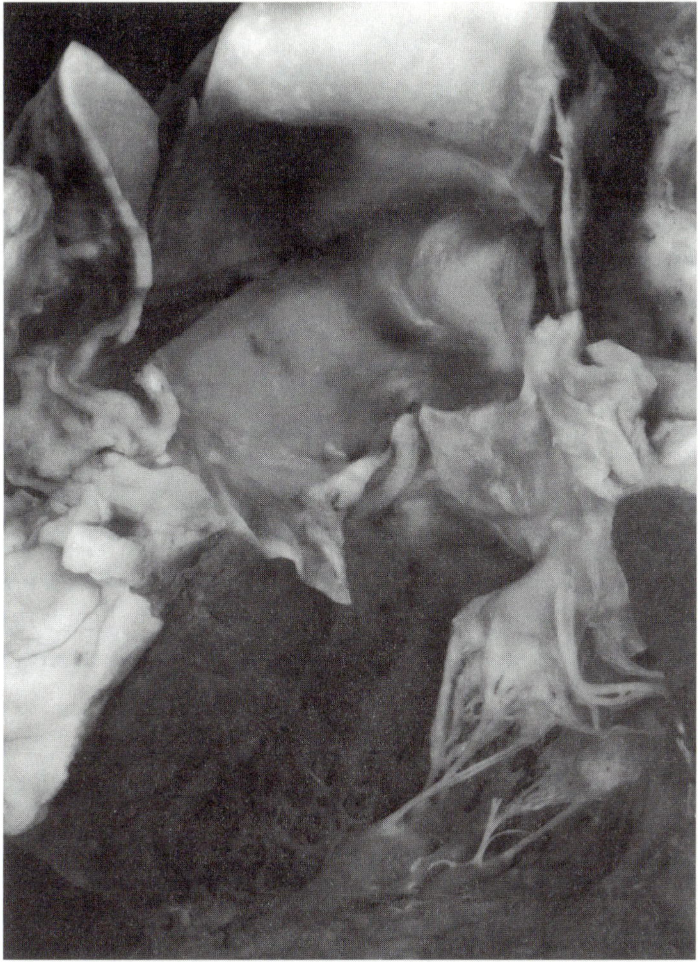

Fig. 1. The opened left ventricle and ascending aorta of a patient with Marfan syndrome. There is a large transverse tear in the ascending aorta, a few centimeters above the aortic valve, leading into an extensive dissecting hematoma with rupture and cardiac tamponade.

rupture often leads to cardiac tamponade and sudden death. Since there are no clinical signs or symptoms that will predict the onset of aortic wall rupture, other than excessive dilation of the ascending aorta or its root, careful follow-up of patients known to have Marfan syndrome is mandatory and preventive surgery is often indicated.

The histopathology of the aortic wall is characterized by widespread fragmentation of the elastin component, although its severity may vary considerably from one site to another. The elastin fibers are often thin and there appears to be a paucity of secondary elastin laminae within the structural units. The elastin frag-

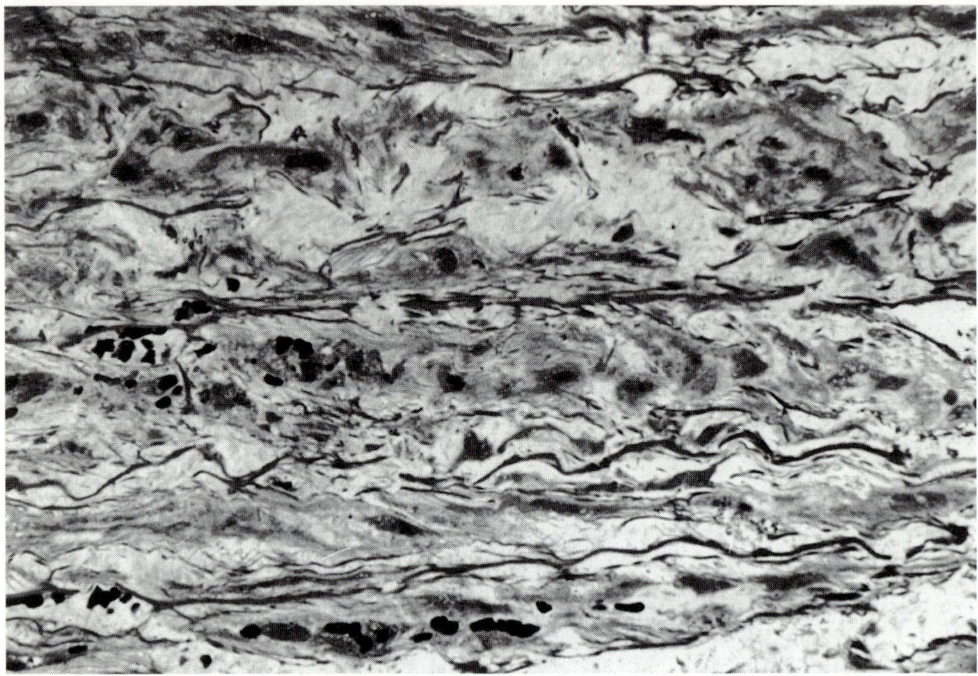

Fig. 2. Light microscopical picture of the aortic wall in a patient with Marfan syndrome. The elastin lamellae are thin and fragmented. Smooth muscle cells have a disorderly arrangement and pooling of extracellular matrix components has occurred. Toluidine blue stain.

mentation (Fig. 2) is accompanied by prominence of vascular smooth muscle cells, often with an almost chaotic arrangement, apparently no longer aligned by the presence of the periluminal elastin lamellae. In addition, mucoid pools occur, always at sites with excessive elastin fragmentation and apparent degeneration of smooth muscle cells. Electron microscopic studies of the aortic wall in patients with Marfan syndrome in part confirm the results obtained with light microscopic studies (Fig. 3). However, areas with pertinent deficiency of elastin fibers may alternate with areas in which distinct elastin components are present, almost as in a normal aorta. It thus appears that heterogeneity of elastin deficiency is the rule rather than the exception. These studies unequivocally demonstrate that a deficiency in the genetic coding for fibrillin may be the underlying molecular genetic fault, but it does not provide an adequate explanation for the morphologic findings in the aortic wall in these patients.

The histopathology of the aortic valves in patients with Marfan syndrome and aortic valve regurgitation is often remarkable. The valves show a basically normal structure, without excessive fragmentation of the elastin component or excessive increase of the mucoid layer, as expected from the basic defect. Instead, a large proportion of these valves have a normal light microscopic appearance, although with secondary effects that relate to the long-lasting regurgitant flow. These changes mainly affect the free edge of the valve leaflets and are composed of concentric layering of collagen fibers mixed with glycosaminoglycans.

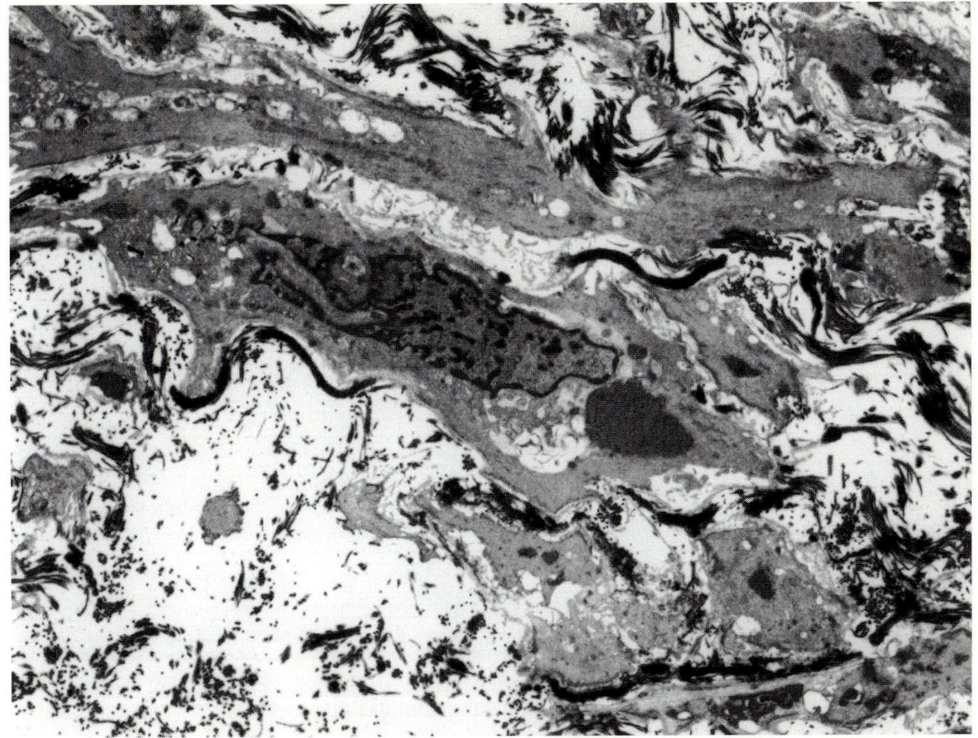

Fig. 3. Electron microscopical detail of the wall of the ascending aorta in a patient with Marfan syndrome. The elastin fibrils are thin and fragmented. The smooth muscle cell present does not reveal abnormal features. The "empty" spaces relate to the pools of extracellular matrix components seen in the light microscopical pictures (see Fig. 2) and, when specifically stained, contain proteoglycans.

Mitral valve pathology

The mitral valve, once affected as part of Marfan syndrome shows diffuse floppiness of the mitral valve leaflets associated with excessive dilation of the valve annulus (Fig. 4). The histopathology of these valves thus show a marked degenerative process of the supportive tissues, which in the valve leaflets proper is manifest as pooling of glycosaminoglycans often with apparent destruction of the fibrous layers of the leaflet. Spontaneous rupture of chords is a common phenomenon, which may cause sudden onset of severe mitral valve regurgitation and left heart failure.

Additional sequelae

Apart from the major conditions described above, arteries and veins, of both large and smaller caliber, may be affected also. The pathology alluded to above may render the patient prone to develop infectious endocarditis. This applies in particu-

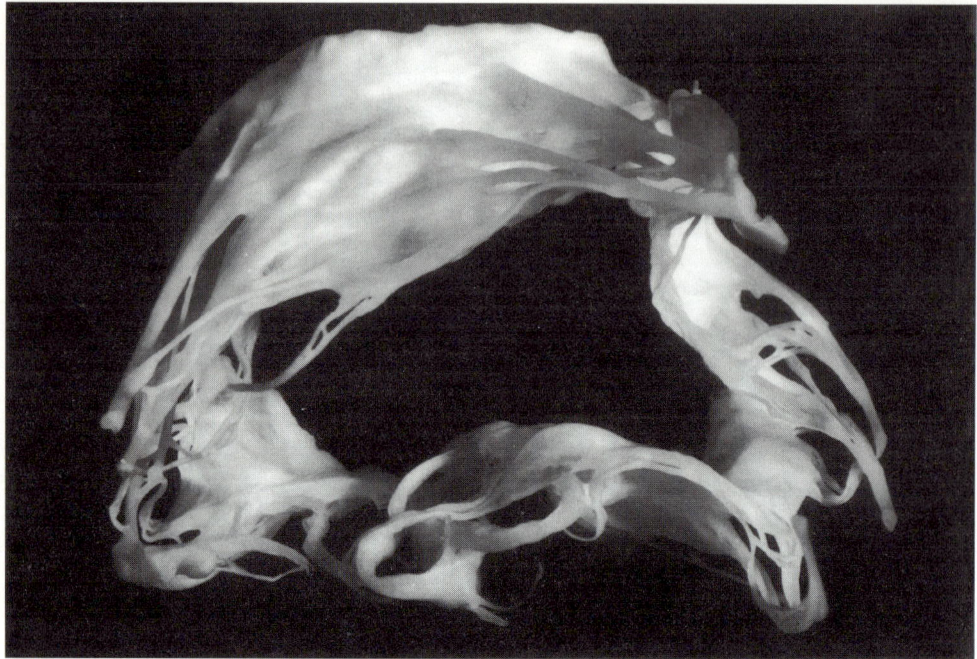

Fig. 4. Ventricular aspect of a surgically resected floppy mitral valve in a patient with Marfan syndrome. Note the excessive circumference indicating annular dilation.

lar to the aortic and mitral valves, where the basic defect leading to valve regurgitation also produces secondary changes known to play a role as a nidus for infection. Furthermore, the affected aortic and mitral valves may enhance additional degenerative changes such as chordal rupture and annular calcifications. However, within the setting of the major catastrophes that jeopardize the lives of patients with Marfan syndrome these additional changes are of little clinical relevance.

Conclusions

The cardiovascular manifestations of Marfan disease are frequent, affect the ascending aorta, aortic root and aortic valve as well as the mitral valve, and relate to the underlying defect in the supportive tissues. Although the molecular genetic basis for Marfan syndrome has been rooted firmly, it also became apparent that other mutations may occur causing disease processes related to classic Marfan syndrome but not encompassing the full phenotypic spectrum. It is of interest, therefore, that the histopathology, both at the light- and electron microscopic level, reveals heterogeneity and certainly is not characterized by the uniform absence of the elastin components. Further, integration between histopathologic observations, preferably with the use of immuno-electron microscopy, and molecular genetics seems mandatory to provide a better understanding of pathogenesis.

References

1. Godfrey M, Menashe V, Weleber RG, Koler RD, Bigley RH, Lovrien E, Zonana J, Hollister DW (1990) Cosegration of elastin-associated microfibrillar abnormalities with the Marfan phenotype in families. Am J Hum Genet 46: 652-660
2. Hollister DW, Godfrey M, Sakai LY, Pyeritz RE (1990) Immunohistologic abnormalities of the microfibrillar-fiber system in the Marfan syndrome. N Engl J Med 323: 152-159
3. Kainulainen K, Pulkkinen L, Savolainen A, Kaitila I, Peltonen L (1990) Location on chromosome 15 of the gene defect causing Marfan syndrome. N Engl J Med 323: 935-939
4. McKusick VA (1955) The cardiovascular aspects of Marfan's syndrome: a heritable disorder of connective tissue. Circulation 11: 321-342
5. Pyeritz RE, McKusick (1979) The Marfan syndrome: diagnosis and management. N Engl J Med 300: 772-777
6. Sakai LY, Keene DR, Engvall E (1986) Fibrillin, a new 350-kD glycoprotein is a component of extracellular microfibrils. J Cell Biol 103: 2499-2509

Author's address:
A. E. Becker, M.D.
Professor of Pathology
University of Amsterdam, Academy Medical Center
Meibergdreef 9
1105 AZ Amsterdam Zuidoost, The Netherlands

Relevance of cystic medial degeneration in cardiac surgery

G. Fraedrich, Ch. Ihling[1], H. E. Schaefer[1], and V. Schlosser

Department of Cardiovascular Surgery and Institute of Pathology[1], University Clinic, Freiburg, FRG

Whereas the etiology of the majority of aneurysms is in nearly all cases atherosclerotic, degeneration of the aortic wall is often responsible for dilating or dissecting diseases of the thoracic aorta (4, 7). Thus, connective tissue disorders involving either elastic tissue degeneration or disturbed collagen synthesis are widely associated with an increased fragility of the aortic wall, as encountered with degenerative tissue abnormalities, in particular in patients with Marfan syndrome (1, 3).

However, these morphological descriptions of cystic medial degeneration are even encountered as coincidental findings in subjectively stable aortic wall conditions. On the other hand, a conspicuous fragility of the aortic tissue does often not correlate to histological disorders (5, 8, 9, 11).

In order to substantiate this experience, we routinely examined 1900 biopsies from the aortic wall in patients undergoing different open-heart procedures. The different diseases as well as the intraoperative findings were compared to the histological results.

Cystic medial degeneration of different extent was found in 97 (or 5.1%) of the aortic wall specimens with an increasing frequency in patients undergoing coronary artery bypass grafting, aortic wall replacement, and repair of traumatic aneurysm or coarctation. As to be expected, in about 79% of the patients operated for aortic dissection cystic medial degeneration was found (Table 1).

With regard to the underlying diagnosis, cystic medial degeneration was suspected preoperatively in most of the patients with thoracic aortic aneurysm or dissection, and intraoperatively in three-fourths of the patients undergoing aortic valve replacement with an increased aortic wall friability. However, in 41% of the cases, the histological description of cystic medial degeneration was purely coincidental (Table 2).

The biopsies were fixed with formalin, embedded and sectioned in paraffin blocks, and than examined with three stains, Alcian-blue, Hematoxylin, and Elastica-van-Gieson. The pathomorphology of cystic medial degeneration was classified into three different degrees:

I) small amount of mucoid substances;

II) storage of mucopolysaccharides, isolated cystic necroses;

III) large amount of mucoid substances, spreading cystic necroses, so-called type Gsell-Erdheim

When comparing the histological grading to the underlying disease, there was no correlation between the morphological degree of cystic medial necrosis and the surgical suspicion of medial degeneration (Table 3).

Although there was a slight correlation to the grade of cystic medial degeneration in those cases where aortic wall friability was of intraoperative importance, in 81%

Table 1: Occurrence of cystic medial degeneration Histologic findings in 1,900 aortic biopsies

Surgery	n	CMD	%
Coronary	1,350	34	2.5
Aortic valve	350	17	4.9
Aortic rupture	16	1	6.3
Coarctation	110	8	7.3
Thor. aortic aneur.	36	7	19.4
Aortic dissection	38	30	78.9
All biopsies	1,900	97	5.1

Table 2. Suspicion of cystic medial degeneration

Surgery	preop (%)	intraop (%)	coincid (%)
Thor. aneu/diss	28 (75.7)	6 (16.2)	3 (8.1)
Aortic valve	4 (23.5)	13 (76.5)	–
Aortic rupture	1 (100)	–	–
Coarctation	–	–	8 (100)
Coronary	–	5 (14.7)	29 (85.3)
All	33 (34.0)	24 (24.8)	40 (41.2)

Table 3. Suspicion of cystic medial degeneration

	preop (%)	intraop (%)	coincid (%)
Grade I	17 (36.2)	12 (25.5)	18 (38.3)
Grade II	7 (22.6)	5 (16.1)	19 (61.3)
Grade III	9 (47.4)	7 (36.8)	3 (15.8)
All biopsies	33 (34.0)	24 (24.8)	40 (41.2)

Table 4. Intraoperative relevance of cystic medial degeneration

	yes (%)	no (%)	n
Grade I	5 (10.6)	42 (89.4)	47
Grade II	6 (19.4)	25 (80.6)	31
Grade III	7 (36.8)	12 (63.2)	19
All biopsies	18 (18.6)	79 (81.4)	97

of all cases the pathomorphology of the aorta had no surgical relevance. In particular, extremely reduced aortic tissue strength did not correlate to the morphological degree of medial degeneration (Table 4).

To, summarize our study, we could observe cystic medial degeneration of different degree with about 5% of routinely examined aortic biopsies, and that occured significantly more frequently with thoracic aortic aneurysm and dissection. However, there seems to be no obvious correlation between the intraoperatively ob-

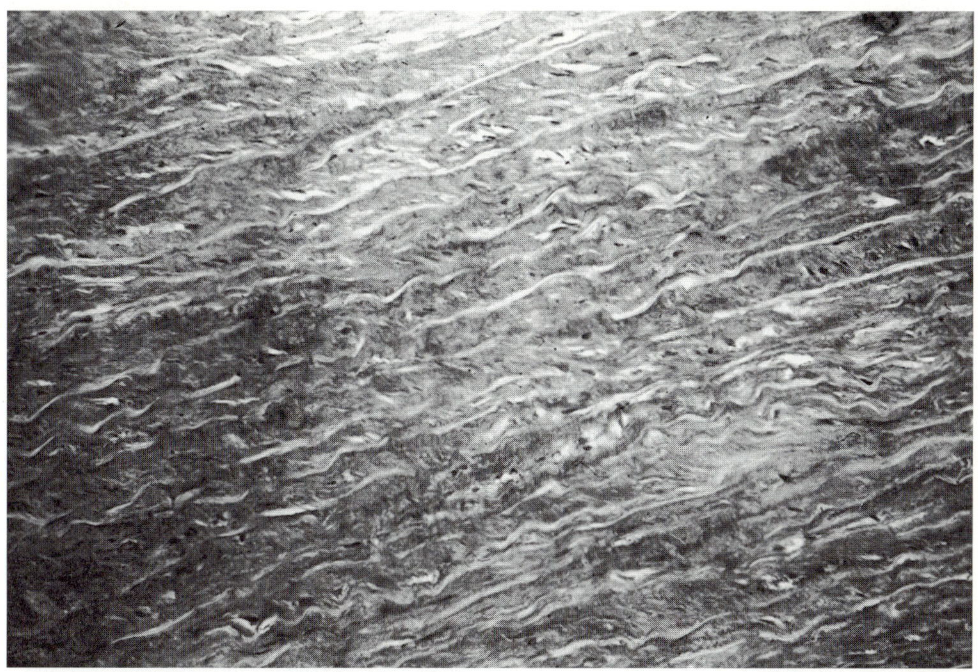

Fig. 1. Small amount of basophile mucoid substances, arranged like clouds in the media, classified as slight alteration of the aortic wall (Alcian-blue strain 10x).

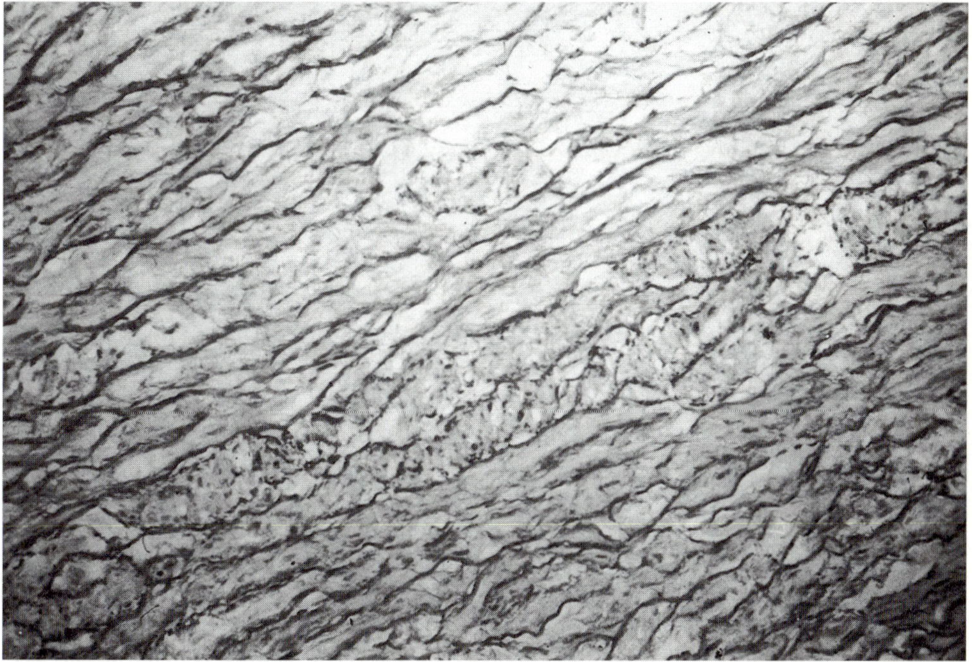

Fig. 2. Broken elastic fibers within small cysts, classified as moderate changes (Elastica-van-Gieson stain 20x).

Table 5. Aortic dissection. Primary etiologic factors (congenital)

- Connective tissue disorders:
  (elastic tissue/collagen synthesis)
  - ► Marfan syndrome
  - ► Ehlers-Danlos' syndrome
  - ► Menke's syndrome
  - ► Turner's syndrome
- Congenital heart disease
  - ► Coarctation
  - ► Bicuspid aortic valve

Table 6. Aortic dissection. Secondary etiologic factors (acquired)

- Hypertension (aortic wall tension)
- Atherosclerosis (atrophy of smooth muscle cells)
- Infection (rheumatic or syphilitic)
- Endocrinologic factors (pregnancy)
- Alimentary factors (copper deficiency)
- Thoracic trauma (deceleration)

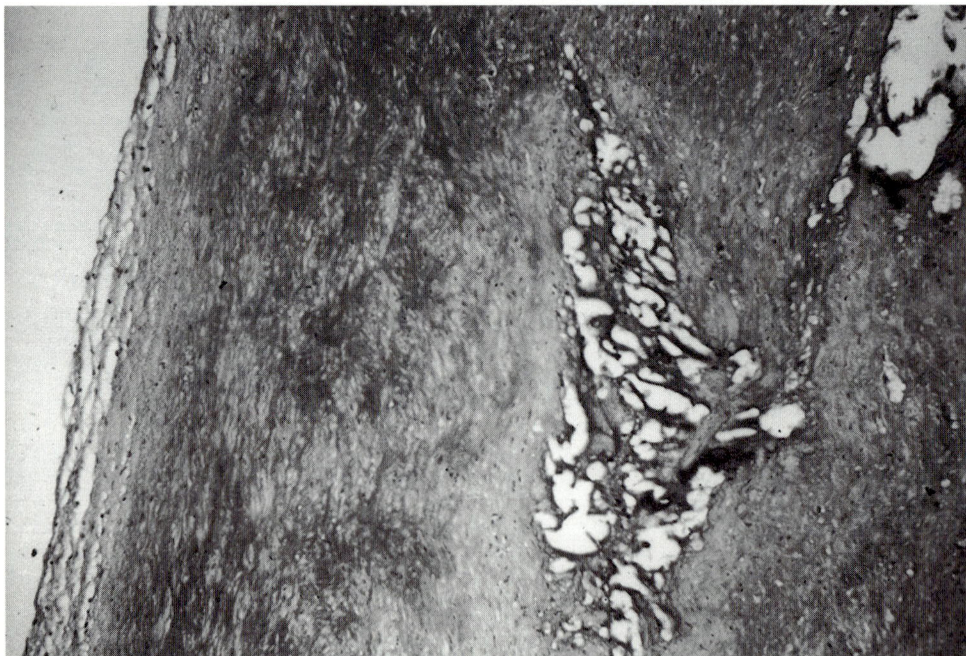

Fig. 3. The continuity of the elastic fibers disappeared and elastic detritus is found within large cyst-like spaces, classified as cystic medial necrosis, of the type Gsell-Erdheim (Alcian-blue stain 10x).

served aortic wall friability and the morphological degree of cystic medial degeneration – and the prognostic relevance of these histological findings seems to be of negligible importance (10).

Therefore, additional etiological factors might contribute to an increased aortic wall fragility, and we propose the pathogenesis mentioned in Tables 5 and 6:

Beside congenital factors (often summarized as cystic medial necrosis) that are encountered particularly in patients with connective tissue abnormalities – like in Marfan syndrome (6) – acquired factors might play an additional role in the etiology of aortic dissection. These secondary factors can presumably explain why about 60% of aortic dissections occur in male patients older than 40 years (2, 5, 8, 9).

References

1. Anagustopoulos CE (1975) Acute aortic dissections. Univ Parc Press, Baltimore, London, Tokyo
2. Carlson RS, Lillehei CW, Edwards JE (1970) Cystic media necrosis of ascending aorta in relation to age and hypertension. Am J Cardiol 25: 411
3. Klima JE (1983) Medianecrosis as cause of dissecting aortic aneurysm. Human Pathol 14: 810
4. Larsone W, Edwards WD (1984) Risk factors for aortic dissections: A necropsy study on 161 cases. Am J Cardiol 53: 849
5. Leu HJ, Schneider J, Oertli Ch, Hofmann H, Walter M (1978) Die mukoide Degeneration der Aorta. Vasa 7: 218
6. Moore HC (1965) Marfan syndrome, dissecting aneurysm of the aorta and pregnancy. J Clin Path 18: 277
7. Roberts WC (1981) Aortic dissection: Anatomy, consequences and causes. Amer Heart J 101: 195
8. Schaefer HE (1990) Morphologische Gesichtspunkte bei Aneurysmen und Dissektionen der thorakalen Aorta. In: Schlosser V, Fraedrich G (eds) Aneurysmen der thorakalen Aorta. Diagnose und Therapie, pp 3–17. Steinkopff Verlag, Darmstadt
9. Schlatmann TJM, Becker AC (1977) Pathogenesis of dissecting aneurysms of the aorta. Comparative histopathologic study of significance of medial changes. Amer J Cardiol 39: 13
10. Schlosser V, Knapp I, Schaefer HE (1987) Vergleichende klinisch-morphologische Untersuchungen zur Bedeutung der zystischen Medianekrose in der kardiovaskulären Chirurgie. Vasa 16: 40
11. Spillner G, Mittermaier Ch, Schlosser V (1978) Die Bedeutung der zystischen Media-Nekrose von Aorta und großen Arterien. Thoraxchir 26: 20

Authors' address:
Priv.-Doz. Dr. G. Fraedrich
Abteilung Herz- und Gefäßchirurgie
Chirurgische Universitätsklinik
Hugstetter Straße 55
79106 Freiburg im Breisgau, FRG

Surgical therapy for Marfan Syndrome – Then and now

H. H. Bentall

Emeritus Professor of Cardiac Surgery, Royal Postgraduate Medical School, University of London, England

Dr. Hetzer had asked me to report briefly on the history of operating for Marfan syndrome. This is a rather gloomy subject!

One case report is particularly illustrative. A male patient, aged 35 years, presented at Hammersmith Hospital in October 1966, was our first surgical patient with this syndrome (2, 7).

Plain x-ray of his chest (Fig. 1) showed slight dilatation of the aortic root and a slightly enlarged left ventricle.

In the angiocardiogram, however (Fig. 2), these features were obviously more severe and there was clear evidence of aortic regurgitation. He had presented with increasing dyspnea and inability to work and was recommended for operation.

Thinking of our own experience of wrapping procedures and of the plication operation of Bahnson (1) in which, in 1954, a vast side-clamp was used to reduce the size of the aortic aneurysm but did nothing for the valve regurgitation, it became clear that a more aggressive approach was required.

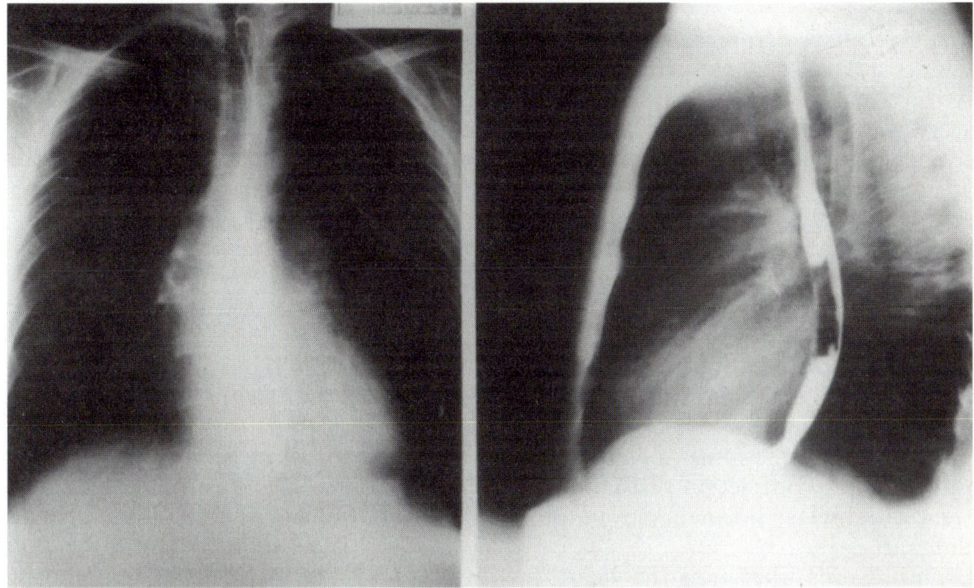

Fig. 1. First patient – Chest film

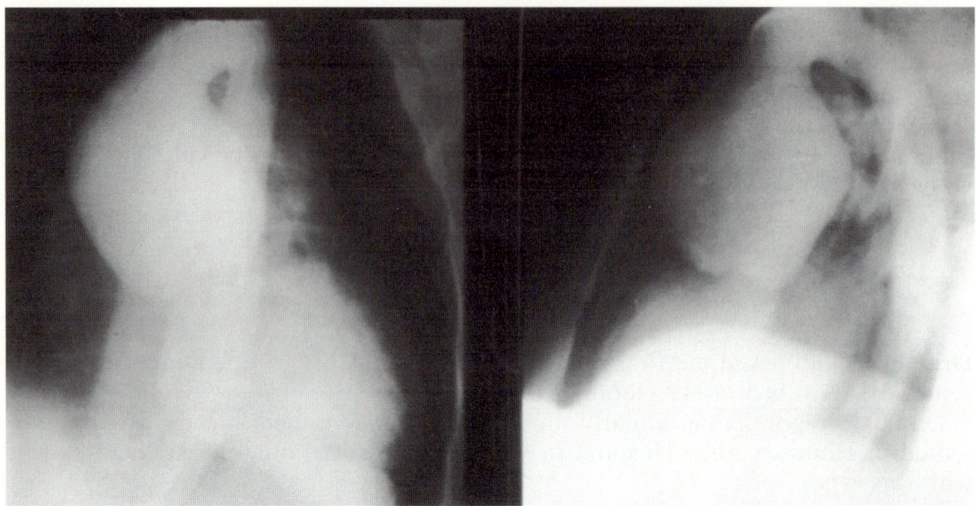

Fig. 2. Angiocardiogram.

The procedure of Wheat (9) in 1964, replaced the aortic valve and grafted the aorta, but left the thin aortic sinuses to be united to the cloth graft; this was not satisfactory as leakage was still a real problem which contributed to mortality.

Bloodwell, Hallman and Cooley (3) showed in 1965, that the caudal displacement of the heart sometimes permitted excision of the aneurysm and performance of direct anastomosis of the aorta to the sinuses or of a similar procedure using a short graft. The results were similar to those of Wheat for similar reasons.

The Operation – November 1966

At the time I had to operate on the patient described, as can be seen in Fig. 3, there was the characteristic avascular area on the front of the aortic aneurysm, strangely enough, not the area through which rupture usually occurs. With the aorta opened (Fig. 4) and the coronary arteries catheterized the heart beats slowly at a temperature of 30 °C. The first sutures have been placed in the aortic "ring" and the mitral leaflets can be seen. On a side table a composite graft was prepared using a Starr-Edwards 1260 valve (Fig. 5). (Commercial composite grafts were of course not available in 1966; in fact, this was the first occasion that such a graft was described).

The composite graft was then sewn by the double-armed interrupted sutures, slid into place (Fig. 6), and holes cut for the left (Fig. 7) and right (Fig. 8) coronary arterial anastomoses. The coronary perfusion was stopped temporarily and replaced through the lumen of the graft and through a small incision in the anterior wall to allow completion of the upper aortic anastomosis. The coronary catheters were withdrawn, the aneurysm tailored (Fig. 9), and the aortic wall closed around the graft.

During this operation the heart was arrested by electrical fibrillation during opening of the aorta, followed by insertion of catheters for coronary perfusion and

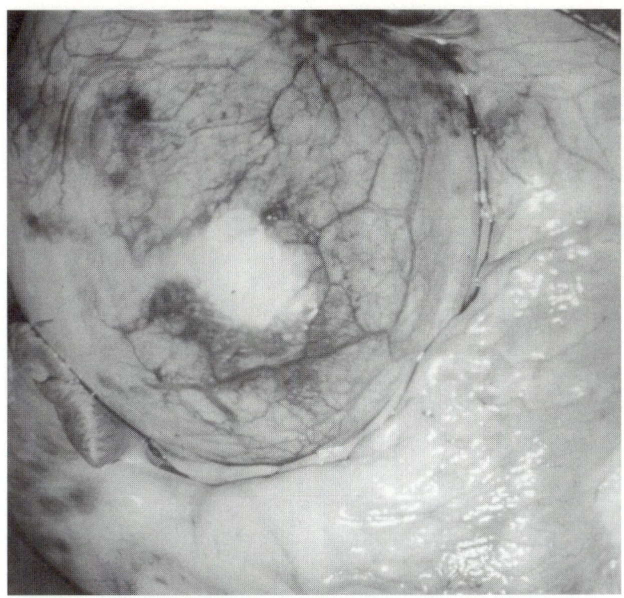

Fig. 3. Aneurysm exposed through median sternotomy.

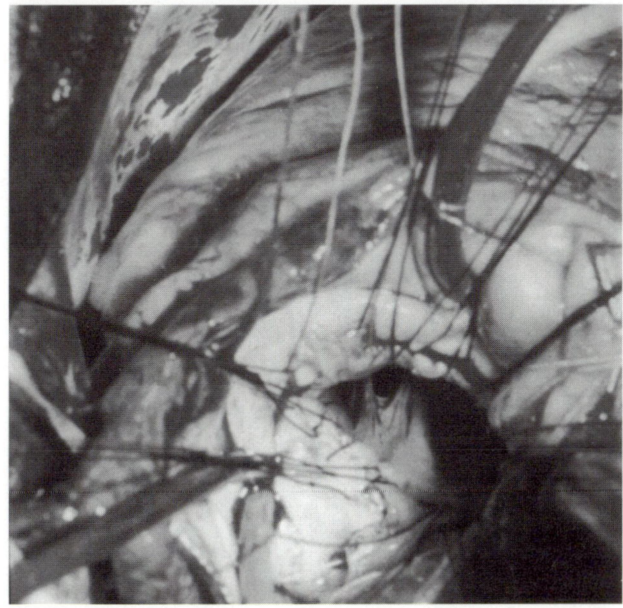

Fig. 4. Aorta open – Coronary arteries catheterized for perfusion.

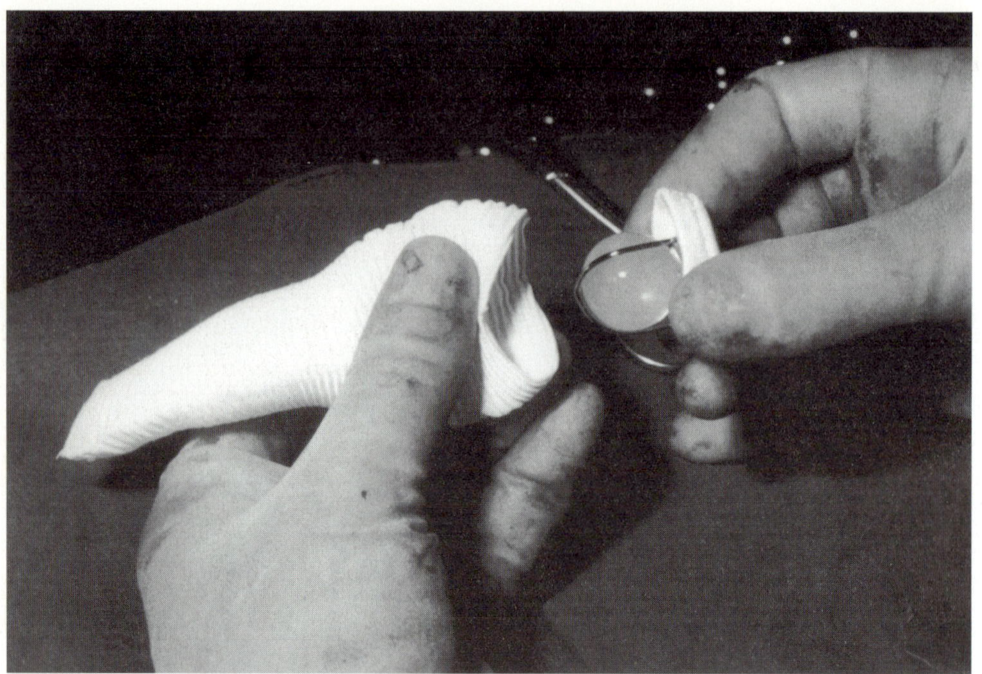

Fig. 5. Composite graft prepared.

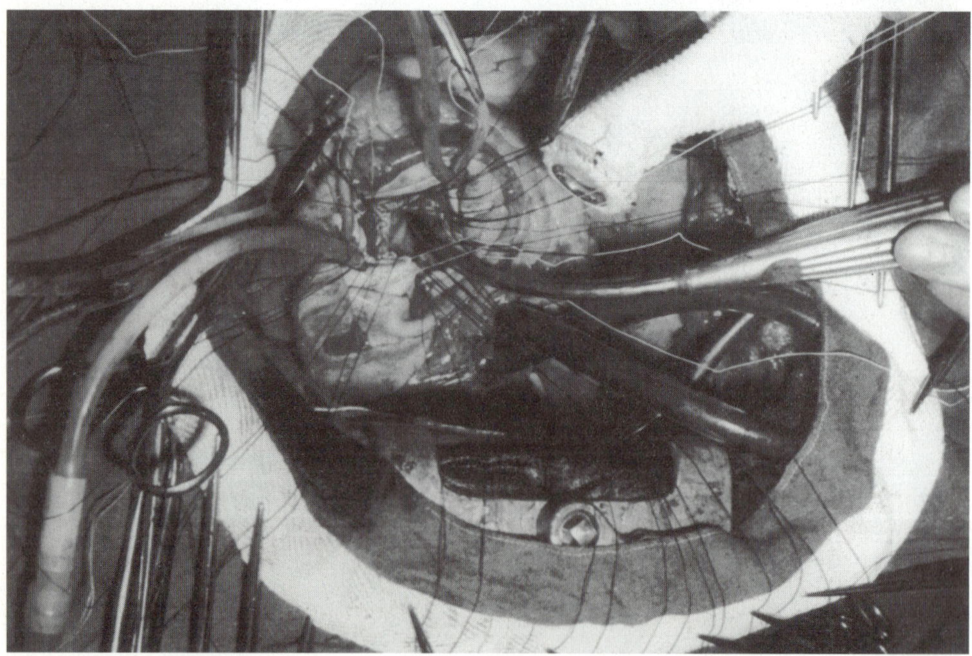

Fig. 6. Placing of graft.

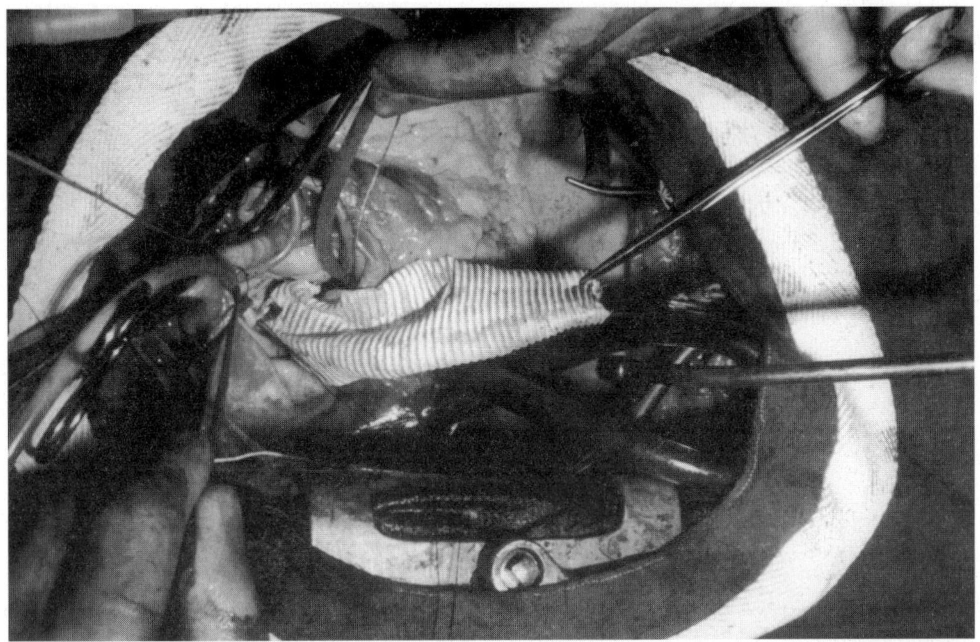

Fig. 7. Cutting hole for left coronary anastomosis.

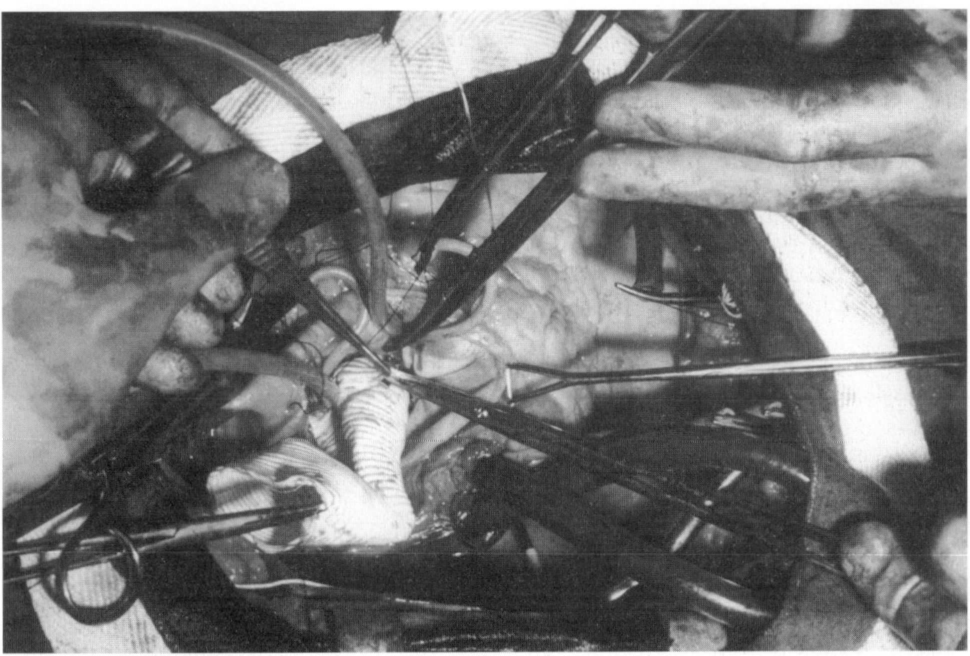

Fig. 8. Cutting hole for right coronary anastomosis.

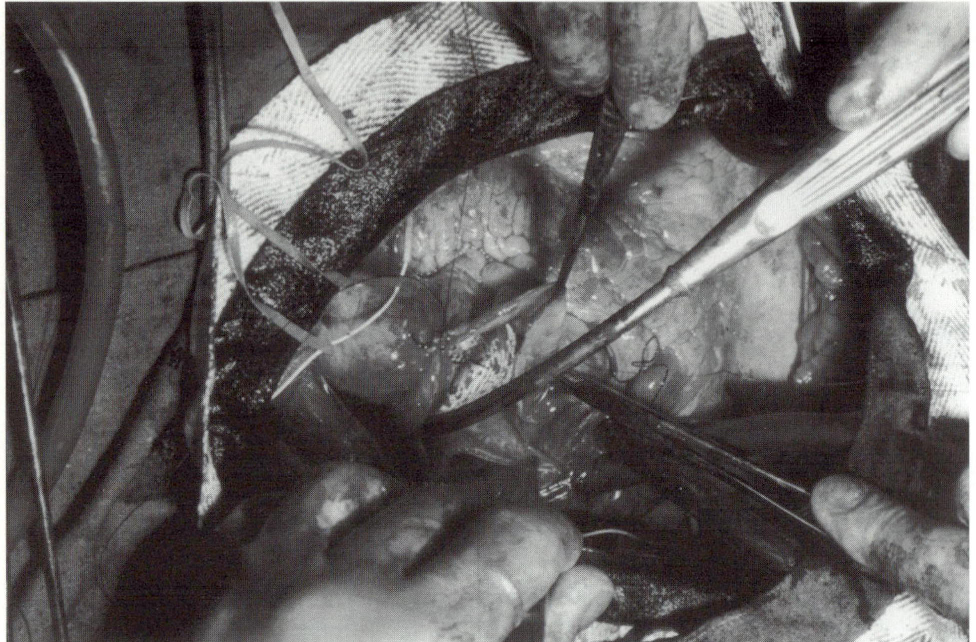

Fig. 9. Aneurysm tailored and being closed around graft.

for their removal and closure of the aorta. For the remainder of the intracardiac procedure the heart was allowed to beat. Rewarming followed closure. This patient made an uninterrupted recovery but died 8 years later from a ruptured dissection 4 cms down his left coronary artery, which was apparently not associated with the anastomosis.

Bleeding through the aortic graft was always a potential problem. Initially, we used a Teflon graft but changed to Dacron as it became available. This permitted use of the actual cautery to cut the hole for the coronary artery (Fig. 10), producing a hole with a non-fraying edge and a sounder union.

Discussion

The original mortality in my own experience was 10%. That was during the learning phase. The results of Gott (Table 1) show the astonishing mortality of 1·4% for his first 140 patients.

This is the only series in the world of all Marfan patients; there were no deaths in the 125 elective cases and 2 deaths of the 15 emergency repairs, both of whom had suffered ruptured aneurysm with tamponade and one of whom was moribund on arrival.

Gott used a "tight" wrap of the graft after trimming the aortic wall (as we had originally described), in his first 87 patients and ,subsequently, a "loose" wrap combined with preclotting of the Dacron graft with 25% albumin as suggested by Kouchoukos (6). This paper reported the etiology, operations, and results in 168

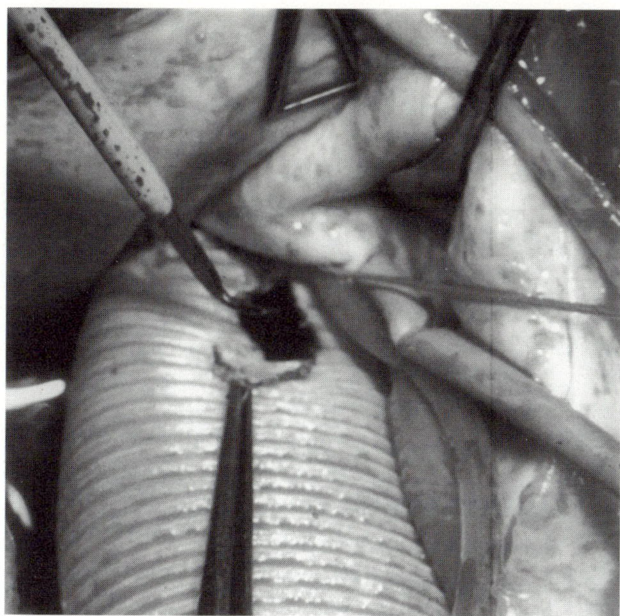

Fig. 10. Method of cutting hole in Dacron graft using actual cautery – a later patient.

patients, in his own experience (Table 2), showing an 18% incidence of Marfan syndrome in units not having a special referral practice for the investigation and medical and surgical treatment of this syndrome, as does Johns Hopkins Hospital in Baltimore. Both authors conclude that the "loose" wrap gives better long-term results than the "tight" wrap.

The excellent long-term results in both of these series showed, however, that the serious complication of prosthetic endocarditis occurred in 6 of 138 survivors (4·35%) with 3 deaths, reported by Gott, and in 7 of 163 survivors (4·35%) with 4 deaths reported by Kouchoukos. Neither author discussed prophylaxis of

Table 1. Aortic root replacement for Marfan syndrome

The Baltimore Experience	
140 Patients had composite graft similar to that described by Bentall and de Bono 1968.	
125 Elective operations – No hospital deaths.	
15 Emergency operations – 2 hospital deaths, both admitted with cardiac tamponade, one moribund on admission.	
"Tight" wrap in first 87 patients – "Loose" wrap since.	
Total hospital mortality – 2 deaths – 1.4%	
Major late complication –	Endocarditis – 6 patients (4 · 35%) 3 treated successfully 3 died.

Ref. (6) Gott et al., 1992.

Table 2. Aortic root replacement

Sixteen-year experience

Division of Cardiothoracic Surgery, Department of Surgery, Washington University School of Medicine, St. Louis, Missouri.

168 Patients

30 Clinical Marfan's

84 Annulo-aortic ectasia
54 Aortic dissection > 28 had both.

Inclusion/"Tight" wrap in first 105 patients –
Open/"Loose" wrap with albumin 25% preclotted graft since.

Endocarditis – 7 patients (4 · 35%)
3 treated successfully
4 died.

endocarditis. Although the evidence is as yet incomplete there is good reason to believe that the use of large dose parenteral antibiotics before and after invasive procedures such a dental surgery (8), urinary catheterization or treatment of infections may reduce the incidence of endocarditis in these vulnerable patients (5).

Conclusion

It seems unlikely that the medical and surgical skills achieved by the Baltimore group which have resulted in a hospital mortality of 1·4% for all comers with Marfan syndrome will be bettered or even easily equaled. Modern techniques of myocardial protection are now well standardized. Some progress is to be made by improvement in the materials used for both valves and conduit in the prevention of thrombosis, and by encouragement of healing and by the discouragement of infection.

In the longer term, vigorous continuous research into the molecular biology of the underlying disease and its genetics could lead to its prevention and eventually to treatment of the biological defect.

References

1. Bahnson HT, Nelson AR (1956) Cystic medial necrosis as a cause of localized aortic aneurysms amenable to surgical treatment. Ann Surg 144: 519–529
2. Bentall HH, de Bono A (1968) A technique for complete replacement of the ascending aorta. Thorax 23: 338–339
3. Bloodwell RD, Hallman GL, Cooley DA (1966) Aneurysm of the ascending aorta with aortic valvular insufficiency. Arch Surg 92: 588–599
4. Fang G, Keys TF, Gentry LO, et al. (1993) Prosthetic valve endocarditis resulting from nosocomial bacteremia. Ann Intern Med 119: 560–567
5. Gott VL, Cameron DE, Pyeritz RE, Reitz BA (1992) The marfan syndrome. Chest Surg Clin of N Amer 2: 425–437
6. Kouchoukos NT, Wareing TH, Murphy SF, Perrillo JB (1991) Sixteen-year experience with aortic root replacement. Ann Surg 214: 308–318

7. Saunders KB, Bentall HH (1967) Aneurysm of the aortic root with gross aortic incompetence: Successful surgical correction. Proc Roy Soc Med 60: 726–727
8. Simmons NA, Ball AP, Cawson RA, et al (1992) Dental prophylaxis for endocarditis, Letter, Lancet 340: 1353
9. Wheat MW Jr, Wilson JR, Bartley TD (1964) Successful replacement of the entire ascending aorta and aortic valve JAMA 188: 717

Author's address:
Prof. H. H. Bentall, FRCS
Pyt Cottage, Marlow Road,
Henley-on-Thames, Oxon
RG9 2JA. UK

Morning panel session

Moderated by Hugh Bentall and Reed Pyeritz

INBERG: My question is very simple, but I do not think the answer is so simple because it illustrates the diagnostic gray-zone between Marfan syndrome and isolated annuloaortic ectasia. At the moment, we are running a study where 70 patients and their 500 first-degree relatives have been included. Most of them are Marfan patients, but in five of these families the diagnostic criteria for Marfan syndrome as established by Beighton et al. in 1986 were not fulfilled. They only had cardiovascular symptoms such as annuloaortic ectasia or mitral valve prolapse. Many of the first-degree relatives in this group had aortic dilatation. So, my question is whether you think that this is the same disease or a different disease?

PELTONEN: You have excellent family material where this could be proved, or proved not to be true. We have now highly relevant markers, polymorphic intragenic markers, for both fibrillin 15 and fibrillin 5. So, I think we could test your hypothesis for positive to either one of those genes.

BENTALL: It has been about a year since we know a little bit about chromosome 15 and chromosome 5, but there may be other fibrillin genes or genes associated with the expression of fibrillin about which we know nothing as yet. Are there beginning to be indications that other of these genes will be discovered in the next five years or so?

PELTONEN: Yes, there are, even in the Nature issue where the first mutation was reported in a paper by Ramirez' group there was an indication on the third fibrillin gene on chromosome 17. This particular gene has turned out to be a cloning artefact, but I am quite convinced that we will follow the story of the collagen gene family here and we will most probably face a fibrillin gene family in the nearest future. I would like to make an additional comment to Dr. Bentall. You referred to the original Marfan paper which most probably describes a congenital contractural arachnodactyly instead of Marfan syndrome, but what is highly interesting to me is that these syndromes will definitely overlap because the neonatal cases of Marfan syndrome carry highly similar ties in phenotype to CCA, i.e. crumpled ears and contractures. Now, there is definitive evidence that at least some of them are caused by mutations in fib 15. So I am quite sure that we know so little about tissue interaction of these two gene products that at this stage it is impossible to predict the precise consequences at the phenotype level.

BENTALL: I think it terribly important that we record, as surgeons, what it is exactly that we are seeing and not just call them Marfan's. I follow Jesse Edwards, who struggled with this for a long time; he used the term "form-fruste Marfan" which we should now, I am absolutely certain, abandon, just as I am absolutely certain we should abandon the term "medial necrosis". Medial necrosis is not a diagnosis for the surgeon.

BECKER: It is interesting to see that in some surgical series of patients with aortic aneurysms in the list of pathogenetic factors you will find all sorts of funny diagnoses lumped together. Some of those patients, for instance, are identified as having Erdheim's Disease, others will have cystic medial necrosis, others will have medial necrosis, as if these were all sort of different diseases. The important thing is that cystic medial necrosis is something which is very difficult to define. It occurs, as we have shown a long time ago, in increasing degrees with increasing age in basically normal aortas, so it is an age-related phenomenon, and not necessarily linked to a diseased state of that aortic wall. So, you have to be very careful in this respect. For instance, just a historical note, that for many people, Erdheim's Disease is the underlying condition in dissecting aneurysm. Erdheim described two patients in two subsequent papers, neither of them had dissection, but they both had a dilated aorta which ruptured.

PYERITZ: Since we are talking about purity of language and nomenclature, I wonder if we should reconsider the term "annulo-aortic ectasia". Although it is a useful term. We think we know what we are talking about, and yet the annulus rarely dilates. So the annulus is not ectatic. Anton, could you suggest a better term for it?

BECKER: I do not think I could, just off-hand, suggest a better term, but your point is well taken. It is just above the annulus. As Sally very nicely showed from the echo study, the dilation is in the sinus much more than it is at the level of the attachment of the valve leaflets. It has much to do with the way the elastin is anchored to the central fibrous body.

BENTALL: Of course, I agree. Initially it is not a dilatation of the valve annulus. The valve annulus is not dilated until the valve starts leaking. Most of these valve leaflets themselves initially are effectively normal, but the annulus eventually dilates and then you get secondary changes such as Anton showed. However, the term annulo-aortic ectasia is quite a useful one for the surgeon to use until we have a diagnosis. It is not a diagnosis, it is sort of an anatomical description of what the surgeon sees. It is used really much more by surgeons than by physicians and certainly does not apply to infants and young children. Here is a question for Dr. Pyeritz. To the surgeon, isolated annulo-aortic ectasia and Marfan syndrome look absolutely the same. I find it extraordinarily hard to believe that ultimately we will not discover any relationship to fibrillin.

PYERITZ: Certainly many of the families, such as Prof. Inberg showed, who have "annulo-aortic ectasia" also have evidence of a more systemic abnormality of connective tissue. The mitral valve prolapse reflects that. If you look at the entire individual, not just the heart and the aorta, you will find that many of those patients will have very subtle skeletal changes, such as abnormal spinal curvature or pectus. I would emphasize looking at the skin because many of those families will show striae in addition, suggesting that indeed it is a systemic disorder of systemic tissue. It would surprise me not at all to find that many of those autosomal dominant families of annulo-aortic ectasia in fact have a defect of fibrillin 15 or perhaps one of the other macromolecules that compose the microfibril. So, I suspect, Hugh, that this really is a phenotypic continuum that will have some basis in pathology of the microfibril.

BECKER: In my limited experience with isolated annulo-aortic ectasia, the aortic biopsies that I have seen in those patients do not show the changes that I am used to seeing in the type A dissection and in Marfan syndrome.

CHILD (St. George's Hospital, London): At the last meeting of the Marfan Consortium in Portland in August, Diana Milewicz from Texas presented 4 patients who had annulo-aortic ectasia in which she had shown they had fibrillin deficiency using her method of fibroblast culture. These were not familial cases particularly, but I think that if we do a consecutive series of patients with familial dominant annulo-aortic ectasia, we will then be able to see how much overlapping there is with Marfan syndrome. Fibrillin deficiency is a huge category that Marfan syndrome fits right in the middle of, because we have not shown heterogeneity at this point, but rather that there are going to be other dominantly inherited conditions that overlap to a certain extent.

BENTALL: This is the next question for Dr. Pyeritz and Dr. Peltonen to address. There are families with dissection of the aorta unlike the other conditions we have mentioned, but who do not present as Marfan syndrome. So we have to ask ourselves, can we find a relationship between isolated aortic dissection, either familial or sporadic, to that of Marfan?

PYERITZ: My comments would be much the same as the answer to the question about annulo-aortic ectasia. There are clearly autosomal dominant pedigrees of ascending aortic dissection in the absence of Marfan syndrome, and often without much pre-existing aortic dilatation or dilatation of the sinuses. These are very difficult families to manage because of the fear of aortic dissection and, without much in the way of a guide to indicate when a prophylactic Bentall procedure should be performed, because the aortic sinuses are not dilating as they would in Marfan Syndrome. Moreover, some of these families have, again, stretch marks or scoliosis or pectus that might help guide you as to who is affected, but trying to determine the proper time to intervene prophylactically is extremely difficult. Studying them genetically is also difficult because, what we have found is that there generally is one generation affected where there have been a number of siblings or cousins who have died of aortic dissection, maybe a few survivors who have had surgery, but the real issue is, what about the next generation? They may have many children, but you cannot determine phenotypically who is affected because they do not have dilatation. Until you know who is phenotypically affected, you cannot do the genetic-linkage studies that Dr. Peltonen is suggesting, and I would agree, they are very crucial. If you had a genetic marker, then you could advise or reassure the children.

PELTONEN: What I would like to firmly state here is that we are still far from understanding the molecular pathology of Marfan syndrome and we are still further away from that goal in the case of these other disease phenotypes. We should still remember that the defined mutations have not been established in the majority of Marfan cases. There are exciting new findings still appearing, including more fibrillin genes. There is a highly important connective tissue gene recently located in the immediate vicinity of fibrillin 15, on chromosome 15, a lysyl oxidase related gene. I mean there are several things which we do not know even about the trivial Marfan cases, not to even talk about these complex or just-one-feature phenotypes which we are discussing here.

BECKER: I got my interest in this disease because of the pathomorphology you see in elderly patients who develop an acute dissection. What sort of relationship can there be between the change that you find, age-related, and those that occur at such an early stage in Marfan syndrome? It could well be that we are dealing with mutations or something somewhere much later leading to dissections which are sporadic and which have nothing of the phenotype of Marfan syndrome, but basically could lead to the sort of same common denominator that is aortic wall disease.

HETZER: From a clinical standpoint, from a moderately large aortic surgical series that we see here, we see many more dissections in patients who have no stigmata of Marfan, neither from their body nor from their aorta. I would estimate that the ratio between a Marfan-typical dissection and a dissection which has obviously no signs of Marfan is about 1 to 10. I am not aware of any good studies on this topic, but from our series I would say, we have probably seen 300–350 ascending dissections here, and maybe only 35 acute dissections in the Marfan patients.

SINIAWSKI (German Heart Institute Berlin): Is there anything like annulo-mitral ectasia, without aortic involvement which is not far away from Marfan syndrome? Is the so-called floppy mitral valve in patients who have no other stigmata of Marfan syndrome in any way connected with it? From a practical point of view, this does exist, but is there any correlation to pathomorphologic findings?

BECKER: I think we have to be very careful here because in elderly people, mitral valve prolapse can occur and I think it has nothing to do with Marfan syndrome at all. It probably has to do with other factors relating to chordal architecture or wear and tear of the connective tissues, whatever the precise etiology and mechanisms involved. The ectasia of the mitral valve annulus is the mere result of the leakage of the valve. So, I think you have to be extremely careful if you have isolated mitral valve prolapse with annulo-ectasia of the mitral orifice to consider that in the group of Marfan. If that is the case in childhood, I think we may have a different ball game, but I must say I have no experience with isolated mitral valve prolapse in children without other stigmata of Marfan syndrome.

Sir YACOUB: Do we have an explanation why there are so many point mutations and deletions on the fibrillin gene and why do we have so many new cases? Why is it that this gene seems to be unstable and not being edited properly? Do we have an explanation for that? How near are we in producing a transgenic model, and if we are going to have a transgenic model, which mutation would you choose?

PELTONEN: Many of us have been puzzled by the same fact. The general rule for dominant diseases actually is that we are faced mostly by a spectrum of new mutations. If we now exclude these repeat mutations for Dystrophia Myotonica Huntington, [JENS; SOMETHING IS

WRONG/MISSING WITH THIS NEXT SENTENCE] but except for, the same rule seems to hold for osteogenesis imperfecta, the same rule seems to hold for several other diseases. We have tried to calculate the mutation rate per nucleotype in the case of fibrillin gene. I would not think that by any means it exceeds the general mutation rate hitting any gene in human genome. Why we are left with such a spectrum of mutations would rather speak for the fact that there is a hot spot at the DNA level, a somehow sensitive region for mutations in the fibrillin gene. One should also remember that these repeat types of genes perhaps had one ancestor gene consisting only of one EGF repeat. So, these typically are met by deletion mutations of functional domains as often seen in EGF deletion where the whole functional domain is removed. We do not have any solid data to suggest that this would be an exceptional gene. Considering the transgenic animal models where I think Harry Dietz is on his way to establish a transgenic pig which I consider an excellent model, seeing as the whole cardiovascular system of pigs is relatively close to that of man and very well studied. That is one thing which will happen in the nearest future. Also, Ramirez in New York is producing transgenic mice and the mutations he has picked to produce these animals are deletion mutations and, my great personal pleasure is that they are focusing on that what they call the crucial region for neonatals.

BENTALL: This slide shows the result of an in vitro fertilization of a cow who had Marfan syndrome by a normal Jersey bull. There are now some offspring, calves. Is this an appropriate model? Is it a useful model?

PYERITZ: This bovine model arose spontaneously in Idaho. The alert farmer told some veterinarians at the veterinary school in Washington state, namely Cathy Potter and Tom Besser, about it. They have studied it extensively over the past 4 or 5 years. It does appear to be an autosomal dominant trait because they have been able to breed it by superovulating the females before they die. They do not survive pregnancy well, so this has to be done by ex utero techniques and the fertilized eggs then reimplanted. But this does appear to be an excellent model for Marfan syndrome in all of the phenotypic features. The difficulty is in keeping the animals alive long enough to study them. They do appear to have fibrillin abnormalities at the biochemical level. The studies looking at genetic linkage of the fibrillin 15 equivalent in the cow have not yet been successfully done because they have not had the right polymorphisms, but we have every expectation that this would be a good model. There are not that many medical schools that are set up to handle cows, so we think that the miniature pig model is going to be more harmonious with most people's laboratories and budgets.

BENTALL: Transgenic mice obviously are extremely attractive, because they are little and they are inexpensive to feed and keep and so on. Have there been any given the human gene? I know it is obviously just about to happen, or has it happened?

PELTONEN: I think the very first mice exist already but no detailed analysis has been carried out, and, of course, I would like to remind you that in many diseases the transgenic have not turned out to be such a success. I hope all the best for their trial, but you know, after all, the mouse heart and human heart are somewhat different.

Sir YACOUB: Dr. Peltonen and Dr. Pyeritz, have you looked at the effect of the different mutations, deletions on the gene product in expression vectors? Specifically, the rather serious mutation you mentioned, the one which kills people, what does that do in an expression vector?

PELTONEN: Yes, we have tried to express these deletion mutations in vitro. We tried to be very clever in the beginning and express the mini-gene, only the long stretch of EGF repeats, and it did not succeed in producing actual polypeptide chains. So currently we have the whole fibrillin cDNA in the expression vector and those studies have just been initiated, so unfortunately I cannot give you any hard data on those, but yes, definitely this work is underway.

PYERITZ: In Harry Dietz' laboratory, he has been successfully expressing individual EGF motifs, the very short polypeptide and expressing the mutated forms and showing in those systems that the abnormal EGF motif does indeed bind calcium abnormally. One of the functions of the EGF-like motif is to bind ionic calcium. The mutations that are pathologic interfere with that binding. Whether or not they disrupt the secondary structure of the motif, the calcium binding seems to be clearly abnormal. Harry Dietz' group at the Johns Hopkins Hospital, Baltimore, were also showing that the individual mutations interfere with hydroxylation of the key residue, with the aspartyl residue, in the EGF motif so that individual mutations are having specific biochemical effects. No one yet has expressed the entire mutant fibrillin and shown how it interacts with its neighbour, its homologue, in the formation of microfibrils. I think that is certainly the next step, and as Leena says, a lot of people are working toward that goal.

Sir YACOUB: Dr. Becker, you have mentioned the myocardium, the connective tissue framework, the idea of myocardial dysfunction, does the fibrillin gene mutation affect the myocardium through the fibrous "framework of the heart"?

BECKER: The question of whether fibrillin deficiency could affect myocardial functional integrity is quite interesting. At present, the current concept is that the very intricate meshwork of connective tissue that enwraps myocytes and connects bundles of myocytes together has, and that has been shown convincingly, an important role to play in the functional integrity of myocardium. But the main constituents of that are considered collagen types I and III. I know of no study thus far that has looked into any possible contribution of elastin let alone of fibrillin in this context.

PYERITZ: We have done those studies using the monoclonal antibody probes for fibrillin 15 and found a great deal of expression of fibrillin 15 in both cardiac muscle as well as skeletal muscle. I am convinced that some mutations will predispose individuals to a skeletal myopathy, many have very underdeveloped shoulder girdles and evidence of a skeletal myopathy, and some patients have a dilated cardiomyopathy that is well out of proportion to the degree of valvular disease that they have.

BECKER: The chromosome 15, would you relate that specifically to a fibrillin problem in those cases where you have cardiomyopathy?

PYERITZ: We think that cardiomyopathy is related to the abnormal fibrillin present in the extracellular matrix of the muscle fibers.

HETZER: We have seen a few cases of cardiomyopathy in a rather higher percentage than we usually find in a normal population which we related to Marfan syndrome. I would like to ask the panel a very provocative question that came up recently at a research foundation discussion: what is the prospect of gene technological intervention in Marfan patients or Marfan families?

PELTONEN: Taking again analogies in other dominant mutations, for instance, in Dystrophia Myotonica, workers are planning to express the normal allele in excessive amounts and partially cure the disease. I hope it is clear for everybody that for these dominant mutations we always have an unpredictable interference of the mutated allele product to the final microfibril formation. Consequently, we have to know so much more about the whole formation and structure of microfibrils that I would not be at this stage very optimistic concerning, for example, gene therapy or stimulation of overexpression of the healthy allele or even some knock-out trials with antisense RNA which have been suggested. I still think that we have to know so much more of the normal molecular background of fibers and fibrillins.

BENTALL: Dr. Hetzer mentioned dilated cardiomyopathy. Now, it is very important that we avoid confusion at this moment between obstructive cardiomyopathy, which exists as a dominant condition, and which has its gene located on chromosome 15, but which is not in the same lockers as the fibrillin gene, and dilated cardiomyopathy. One was the theoretical possibility of dilatation occurring due to the fibrillin problem, the other is the obstructive cardiomyopathy which is adjacent to it.

Dr. DENG (University of Munster): Based on your prospective trial on β-blockade, Dr. Pyeritz, could you comment on the rationale, the indication, dosage, and mode of monitoring β-blockade.

PYERITZ: The trial is now completed. The rationale was based on animal models, the well-known turkey model of aortic rupture, a mouse model, in vitro systems dating back to the time of Wheat and Palmer in the 1960's. The rationale for using β-blockade was primarily hemodynamic, reducing both the impulse of left ventricular ejection on the sinuses at risk as well as reducing the number of insults, i.e., the number of heart beats, over time. There have been a number of retrospective trials done, retrospective examinations of patients on β-blockade compared to those off. The only randomized trial of which I am aware is one that I started in the late 1970's at Hopkins comparing propranolol to no treatment. That study is now in press in the New England Journal of Medicine. The results were very positive in favour of β-blockade and we continue to believe that β-blockade is useful. We would recommend it for any patient who has any degree of aortic sinus dilatation, no matter how young that patient is. We have perhaps an aggressive viewpoint.

Technical aspects of aortic surgery for Marfan syndrome

C. Cabrol

Hôpital La Pitié, Paris, France

Our total experience of aortic surgery for Marfan syndrome includes 281 patients and covers either true aneurysm or dissections of the ascending aorta, the aortic arch and abdominal aorta.

In the ascending aorta (213 patients), we saw two kinds of lesions : annuloaortic ectasia or supracoronary lesions. In the *supracoronary lesions* (79 patients), surgical treatment was supracoronary aortic replacement. In most of the cases, we used the inclusion technique, replacing most of the ascending aorta alone in seven patients, and in 72 other cases with separate replacement of the aortic valve. We finished by closing the aneurysmal sac connected by a fistula with the right atrial appendage to drain the oozing around the graft.

In annulo aortic ectasia with or without dissection (134 patients), we performed a total replacement of the ascending aorta. The typical angiographic aspect of such disease shows the aortic dilatation starting at the aortic annulus and a severe aortic regurgitation. The typical aspect of the operation is a huge dilatation of the ascending aorta. For the first nine cases, this total replacement of the ascending aorta was performed with a Dacron graft and direct reimplantation of the coronary arteries according to the technique of Bentall and de Bono; in the following cases we used a slight modification of this technique.

This modification consists of placing the valve in the aortic graft 2 cm above the proximal end of the graft, and performing the coronary anastomosis using another Dacron graft. We do not use the usual composite graft because that would require the availability of all suitable sizes for the aortic orifice. By doing so, we were able to use the same size of Dacron graft, 30 mm internal diameter, and for the coronary graft the same 8 mm internal diameter size for all cases. Either a Björk or Medtronic or St. Jude valve was used. We make this composite graft on the operating table by suturing the valve inside the prosthesis 2 cm above the proximal end of the graft. After initiating cardio-pulmonary bypass between two venae caval catheters and a femoral arterial catheter, we clamped the aorta, did the myocardial preservation, and opened the aneurysm longitudinally.

The myocardial preservation was done, in the first half of our cases, by inducing moderate core hypothermia at 30 °C, then topical pericardial hypothermia using saline at 4 °C and crystalloid cardioplegia, usually with St. Thomas solution and lowering the myocardial temperature to 15 °C. For the second half of the cases we used blood cardioplegia and also some moderate core hypothermia. After opening the aneurysmal sac, we excised the aortic valve. We started with anastomosis of the coronary graft on the left coronary orifice with a running 5-0 prolene suture. Then, we performed the proximal aortic graft anastomosis with a running 4-0 prolene suture, and we performed the distal aortic anastomosis the same way, working inside the sac according to the inclusion technique. After that, we performed the anastomosis between the right coronary ostia and the coronary graft using a 5-0 prolene running suture. Finally, a side-to-side anastomosis was done between the coronary graft and the aortic graft. Notice that we never placed the coronary graft behind the aorta, but always in front of it. We closed the sac after resecting the excess tissue and we created a small fistula between the tip of the right atrial appendage and the aortic aneurysmal sac.

When the aneurysm or the dissections involved *the aortic arch* (34 patients), we performed the same technique on the proximal aorta, but we displaced the distal anastomosis in the aortic arch or in the beginning of the descending aorta using the open technique described by Cooley.

Isolated descending thoracic aortic aneurysms were treated with isolated descending thoracic aorta replacement on eight patients for type-B dissection. The aorta was clamped above and below the lesions, opened, and replaced with a Dacron graft. In all these cases and especially when the lesions extended down to the diaghragm, there was a risk of spinal chord ischemia and post-operative paraplegia. Spinal chord protection was obtained using femoro-femoral bypass with the aid of a pump oxygenator, and myocardial and cerebral protection was accomplished by allowing the heart to continue beating in order to ensure the upper body blood circulation.

Whenever possible, a preoperative aortogram was made to try to localize the origin of the Adamkiewicz artery, the main supply of the lower dorsal spinal chord, in order to reimplant on the Dacron graft a part of the posterior wall or the aneurysm where the artery was found to originate.

During surgery of the lesions of the *descending thoracic aorta involving the abdominal aorta,* the main problem was organ protection and concerned the abdominal viscerae and the spinal chord. The lesions seen in 18 patients were classified into two main categories.

Some lesions involved only the upper part of the abdominal aorta but not the distal part of the vessel proximal to its division. They were observed in 15 patients. The procedure usually performed was a bypass exclusion of the diseased aortic segment which, in our experience, was the easiest and simplest procedure; it allowed the aneurysm to thrombose except for the lower part vascularizing abdominal and spinal chord arteries.

Therefore, first an end-to-side distal anastomosis between a Dacron graft and the distal abdominal aorta was performed without any circulatory assistance. Then, under standard cardiopulmonary bypass, moderate hypothermia and low systemic perfusion pressure the proximal descending thoracic aorta was interrupted and closed and the Dacron graft was anastomosed end-to-end to the distal aortic arch, or end-to-side to the ascending aorta.

When the thoraco abdominal aortic aneurysms involved *the entire abdominal aorta,* its branches and the proximal iliac arteries, as observed in three patients we also used the bypass exclusion technique. The distal part of the aortic arch was clamped and a femoro-femoral bypass with a pump oxygenator was set up to protect the spinal chord and the abdominal organ. Then, a distal anastomosis was performed on the two iliac arteries with a bifurcated Dacron graft and a step-by-step retrograde revascularization technique was used to reimplant each abdominal artery on the Dacron graft, one after the other, beginning distally and displacing the clamp of the Dacron graft proximally after each anastomosis. The upper part of the graft was then anastomosed proximally to the aortic arch or ascending aorta as previously described.

When *thoraco abdominal aneurysms included the aortic arch* as we observed in three patients, the surgical procedure started with a distal step-by-step Dacron graft replacement of the abdominal aorta with retrograde reimplantation and revascularization of the abdominal branches on the graft. Then the proximal end of the abdominal Dacron graft was anastomosed end-to-side on the ascending aorta. The brachio cephalic arteries were reimplanted with the aid of a bifurcated Dacron prosthesis anastomosed end-to-side to the proximal part of the abdominal Dacron graft and distally end-to-side to the brachio cephalic trunk and the left carotid artery. Finally, the aorta was closed at the level of the proximal aortic arch according to the bypass exclusion technique we used on all these cases.

In aortic aneurysms including the *entire aorta,* from the aortic valve to the distal abdominal aorta, we had to use all the possible surgical resources: step-by-step replacement, cardiopulmonary bypass with blood cardioplegia, and cold blood carotid artery perfusion or deep hypothermia and total circulatory arrest, as in the four patients with dissecting aneurysms we observed.

The first patient, a 30-year-old woman with Marfan syndrome was operated upon 9 years earlier for dissection of the ascending aorta and had total replacement of the ascending aorta and the aortic valve with a composite graft and coronary arteries reimplantation with a second Dacron graft. At rehospitalization a dissection of the whole aorta with diffuse dilatation of the false channel was discovered. Using a median sternotomy, a median laparotomy, and a bilateral cervical incision, a bifurcated Dacron graft was first inserted into the iliac arteries and was brought up through the diaphragm into the thorax. A second bifurcated graft was implanted end-to-side onto both carotid arteries. Cardiopulmonary bypass was started. Under profound hypothermia (20°C) and total circulatory arrest, the preexisting prosthesis in the ascending aorta was transected at its distal extremity and the distal ascending aorta was closed. The carotid graft was implanted end-to-end to the distal extremity of the composite graft and the Dacron graft coming from the iliac arteries was implanted end-to-side onto the composite graft. Cardiopulmonary bypass was stopped. The right carotid arteries were transected at their origin and sutured. A graft was implanted between the right subclavian artery and the right carotid graft. The same was done on the left side with the left subclavian artery.

A second patient with Marfan syndrome had significant aortic incompetence with a dissection involving the whole aorta, except for the first 2 cm of the ascending aorta. Using a median sternotomy and a median laparotomy, a bifurcated tube graft was implanted onto the iliac arteries and all the abdominal arteries were reimplanted on the graft. Cardiopulmonary bypass was started with moderate hypothermia, cold perfusion of carotid arteries and blood cardioplegia. The supra aortic branches were inserted on the aortic Dacron graft. The ascending aorta was transected 2 cm above the aortic valve. The aortic valve was replaced. The proximal end of the aortic graft was implanted end-to-end onto the proximal section of the ascending aorta. The distal extremity of the ascending aorta was oversewn.

A third patient had the same type of lesion, but the ascending aorta was dissected at the level of the aortic valve. He underwent the same surgical correction for the distal lesions, but for the total replacement of the ascending aorta which was required, we used our usual technique with reimplantation of the coronary arteries with a separate Dacron graft anastomosed side-to-side to the ascending aortic graft.

A fourth patient had undergone surgery for an acute dissection of the ascending aorta 1 month earlier and had a supra coronary graft. The descending thoracic and abdominal aorta were ectatic. Using a median sternotomy and a median laparotomy, a bifurcated graft was inserted onto the iliac arteries and the abdominal branches were reimplanted on it. The graft was brought up into the thorax. Cardiopulmonary bypass was started with moderate hypothermia and myocardial protection was provided by blood cardioplegia.

The ascending aortic graft was excised and the distal ascending aorta was sutured. A second bifurcated graft was anastomosed end-to-end to the proximal part of the ascending aorta. The graft coming from the iliac arteries was anastomosed end-to-side to this bifurcated aortic graft. Cardiopulmonary bypass was stopped. Under continuous electroencephalographic monitoring, the left carotid and brachiocephalic arteries were anastomosed end-to-end to the second bifurcated aortic graft. The left subclavian artery was implanted on the left carotid artery.

Results will first be analyzed in patients with *surgery of ascending aorta.* Although in such patients we performed an associated procedure (mitral repair in one case, mitral valve replacement in six cases, and coronary artery bypass graft in 16 cases), the overall early mortality was 6.3% and the surviving patients were followed up to 11 years. We lost only 12 patients at follow-up. The actuarial survival curve shows a survival rate of 71.7% at 9 years.

In one-third of the patients, we did angiographic control 1 to 5 years after operation. In none of the cases with total replacement we found any aortic insufficiency. In three patients, the right limb of the coronary graft was occluded. The corresponding right coronary artery was a rudimentary one. The angina was moderate and easily controlled by drug treatment. In all other aortic injections it was easy to see the aortic graft and on it the typical aspect of the coronary graft which has a "moustache" appearance. Leaving a clip as a marker on the side-to-side anastomosis between the aortic and the coronary grafts allowed selective injection of the coronary graft, showing in all cases the nice continuation between the graft and the right and the left coronary arteries. We have never seen any aneurysm at the anastomosis site with the coronary arteries.

The late morbidity also concerned three aortic right atrium fistulas. In one case, the fistula was very small and we did not reoperate on the patient. In the other case, the shunt was significant and reoperation was decided 1 year later. It was not necessary to use cardiopulmonary bypass, because on opening the aneurysmal sac, we found a leak in the distal anastomosis of the aortic graft, and we could repair this leak very easily with a suture. On a third patient, a 19-year-old young male, we did a total replacement of the ascending aorta and the aortic valve in our usual manner. Two days after the operation we observed a tremendous shunt through the fistula into the right atrium. On the post-operative angiogram, we demonstrated at the distal aortic anastomosis an acute dissection leaking in the aneurysmal sac, and into the right atrium. We reoperated upon this patient, and we did a successful complementary replacement of the aortic arch. In that case, the right atrial fistula was life-saving.

The main late problem remains to be iterative distal dissection. In 10 patients, we observed such a distal dissection 1 to 8 years after the first operation. In five patients, we did an aortic arch replacement and in one patient a descending thoracic and abdominal aortic replacement.

For lesions of the aortic arch, thoracic descending aorta and abdominal aorta the early surgical mortality is higher by 22–31% and mainly due to hemorrhage and pulmonary insufficiency. Most of the secondary deaths are due to the aneurysmal development of a false channel and to its rupture.

It is thus important that these patients be followed up regularly by CT scanning, color-flow Doppler echography, magnetic resonance imaging and, if necessary, aortography. If the false channel progressively enlarges, it may be necessary to reoperate.

The survival at 9 years varies from 61% for patients treated for aortic arch lesions to 49% for patients with thoracic and/or abdominal lesions and 42% for patients reoperated upon secondarly.

Author's address:
Prof. Dr. Ch. Cabrol
Hopital de la Pitie
Et 83 Pitie Salpetriere
F-75047 Paris
France

The mechanism and prevention of aortic dissection in Marfan syndrome

F. Robicsek, M. Thubrikar

Heineman Medical Research Foundation and The Carolinas Heart Institute at the Carolinas Medical Center, Charlotte, North Carolina, USA

Gradual, continuous dilatation is the sine qua non of aortic dissection

When Marfan published the first report of what came to be known as "Marfan syndrome" in 1896, he emphasized primarily the ocular and skeletal abnormalities (9). The major cardiovascular components of the disease were described by Etter and Baer in 1943 (1, 5). Marfan syndrome occurs in patients who are heterozygous for a mutation that alters one or more components of the extracellular matrix (12, 22). It has been shown that in Marfan syndrome the elastic fibers ordinarily prominent in the aortic media appear disorganized and fragmented. This defect, presumably induced by biochemical changes, renders the aorta susceptible not only to dilatation, but also to dissection (22) which eventually leads to the demise of 90% of those who suffer from this disease.

Dissection is defined as the pathological state in which a tear develops on the inner layer of the aorta and blood enters the aortic wall. This entry seldom occurs between the intima and the media, but usually develops within the media itself or, less frequently, between the media and the adventitia. Thus, with special respect to dissection, the aorta may be compared to a two-ply tube; the inner layer is composed of the intima and part or all of the media and the outer layer is formed of the rest of the media and the adventitia. As blood surges through the tear, it separates the internal and external layers and then propagates centrifugally, although occasionally the dissection extends in both directions or even only proximally. In the course of this process, circulation in the aortic branches may be compromised or, in the case of proximal extension, aortic regurgitation may develop. Re-entry from the false lumen into the true channel can occur at any point. Dissection may end in rupture or, less frequently, it may cause fatal circulatory impairment to vital organs. Depending on its location and underlying pathology, dissection may also enter a chronic state.

The question arises: *Why does dissection develop?*

The integrity of the aortic wall depends on two principal factors: The *holding power* of its components as determined by biochemical and anatomical structure, and the *mural stress* acting upon the anatomical structure and directly related to blood pressure, luminal diameter, and wall thickness. This may be expressed by the standard formula (similar to a modified Laplace formula):

$$S_c = \frac{PR}{T} \text{ and } S_l = \frac{PR}{2T}$$

where S_c is circumferential stress, S_l is longitudinal stress, P is blood pressure (pressure gradient), R is aortic radius, and T is wall thickness. Accordingly, patients who develop aortic dissection may be divided into two major groups: Those with hypertension and those with conditions characterized by inborn weakness of the aortic media (Marfan group).

The common clinical and hemodynamic denominator in these two conditions which predisposes to dissection is *dilatation of the aortic arch,* moderate but always present in hypertension and progressively severe in Marfan syndrome. Therefore, it is logical to accept that aortic dilatation is not only a frequent occurrence in aortic dissection but it is *the precursor to dissection itself.* Furthermore, we postulate that dissection occurs not only in dilated aortas but also only in *dilating* aortas. Aortic dissection would not occur in patients with aortic arch dilatation if further increase in diameter could be prevented.

In hemodynamic terms, a break in the aortic wall occurs whenever the stress exerted upon it (S_c or S_l) exceeds its tensile strength at any point (18). For practical purposes, pressure gradient across the artery wall approximately equals arterial blood pressure (P), which is expressed in dyn. cm^{-2}, while R and T are defined in centimeters.

While abnormal increase in radius (R) is always present in dissection, its *degree* varies. It is usually moderately increased in hypertension and significantly increased in Marfan syndrome. In most cases the changes in radius also will invoke inverse changes in wall thickness (T). Changes in blood pressure (P) occur in reverse in these two conditions, significantly elevated in hypertension but normal in an overwhelming number of cases of Marfan and associated syndromes. Thus, aortic wall stress increases primarily by the pressure-rise in hypertension

$$S_c = \frac{P'R}{T} \text{ and } S_l = \frac{P'R}{2T}$$

and primarily by diameter increase in Marfan,

$$S_c = \frac{PR'}{T} \text{ and } S_l = \frac{PR'}{2T}$$

where P' and R' represent increased pressure and increased radius, respectively.

This progressive dilatation of the ascending aorta in the Marfan patient has been studied by several investigators (13, 16, 22), who found that the enlargement of the ascending aorta usually already manifests in early childhood and begins at the level of the sinuses of Valsalva (16). While on objective measurement the diameter of the ascending aorta, corrected for body surface area, indeed was found to be larger in patients with Marfan syndrome than in control subjects, the diameter of the abdominal aorta in the same group, corrected for body surface area, was not statistically different [8]. This confirms that the brunt of the circulatory consequences of the aortic wall changes in Marfan syndrome are localized to the ascending aorta. Because aortic diameter depends on the distending pressure, but distensibility decreases exponentially as the pressure increases, in Marfan syndrome, where abnormal changes occur in the aortic wall, enlargement of the luman occurs at lower pressures and the limits of distensibility may be reached even at normotensive levels. In a significant share of patients with Marfan syndrome, the dilatation of the ascending aorta will also lead to dilatation of the aortic valvular annulus. Less frequently, aortic regurgitation precedes ascending aortic dilatation, probably because of inborn abnormalities in the aortic cusps (11).

The fact that only a small fraction of hypertensive patients, versus a great share of Marfan patients, develop dissection may be explained by the *relatively limited effect of pressure increase compared to the exponential effect of diameter enlargement upon aortic wall stress.*

As has been stated before, in the process of diminishing wall strength which occurs during dilatation, besides the quantitative factor, i.e., thinning of the vascular wall and decrease of the volume of material forming one unit of the circumference, a qualitative factor, namely, *disruption of the structural integrity of the arterial wall,* also plays an important role. This structural integrity largely depends on the presence of both elastic and collagen fibers in the aortic wall (3). In Marfan syndrome, these fibers are not only absolutely and proportionally decreased by their sparser presence, but also weakened by fragmentation, disorganization, and other degenerative changes (17).

Collagen fibers are aligned circumferentially and the elastin are in an interwoven net. Wolinsky has shown that, within the physiologic pressure range, the collagen bears the tangentially acting forces while the elastic network distributes the stress uniformly throughout the aortic wall (21). It is very likely that the proportions in the sharing of this stress by collagen and elastin varies at different filling pressures. It has been speculated (14, 15) that as the intraaortic pressure increases the increment in mural stress aligns the collagen fibers and the resistance to stressing forces is gradually transferred from elastin to collagen. It has also been noted that the thoracic aorta is about 1.5 times as stiff circumferentially as longitudinally at 100 mmHg internal pressure (2).

Elastin may be extended readily to 250% of its original length (14). Bergel concluded that the difference in behavior between the aorta and other vessels at between 60 and 100 mmHg pressure is due to the great preponderance of elastin over collagen (2:1) found only in the thoracic aorta (2). This parallel arrangement of components implies that the properties of the arterial wall are more directly related to radius than to pressure (2). It is probable that the collagen content of the "inner layer" is relatively lower than that of the "outer layer" and therefore the yield point (tensile strength) of the inner layer is low. Thus, whenever the pressure-stress reaches "the breaking point" the internal layer tears while the outer layer does not.

It is interesting to note that while the thoracic aorta, especially the arch, is so susceptible to dissection, the abdominal aorta is not. The answer may lie in the already-mentioned different tensile strengths of these two segments (7). In his *in vitro* experiments, Bergel found a roughly linear relation between pressure and radius up to 100 to 120 mmHg in the thoracic aorta, but a much steeper increase in modulus in other vessels. Changes in the aortic diameter from diastole to systole are significantly less in the ascending aorta in patients with Marfan syndrome, probably because of the aorta's already overdistended state. A similar relationship, but to a much lesser degree, exists in hypertensive subjects, as well as in patients with coronary artery disease, poststenotic aortic dilatation, and advanced age (15). These changes in circumferential strain are also proportional to the alteration in wall thickness caused by the process of acute dilatation. In other words, besides increase in the radius and/or pressure, *thinning of the arterial wall* is a major factor in stress increase and consequent aortic rupture.

In the example presented by Sumner in 1989, the wall of a blood vessel with an outside diameter of 2 cm and an inside diameter of 1.8 cm and a blood pressure of

150 mmHg would be exposed to a circumferential stress of 8.0 × 10 (12) dyn · cm^{sec-2}. If the artery is aneurysmatically dilated to triple its outside diameter, the 0.2 cm thick arterial wall, not having increased the volume of material in it, will decrease to 0.06 cm in thickness. This will increase the wall stress by a factor of 12 (13).

All of the above considerations relate closely to aortic dissection if the factor wall strength (W_{st}) is replaced by the sum of $W_{sti} + W_{sto}$, i.e., the strength of the inside and outside aortic wall layers. Accordingly, the wall stress, S_c or S_l, may exceed the strength of the inner, but not the outer, layer.

$$S_c \text{ or } S_l > W_{sti} < W_{sto}$$

The marked thinning of the wall which may occur under increasing pressure corresponds to lamellar straightening of the elastin, decreased interlamellar distances and decreased lamellar thickness. However, interlamellar distances decrease more than lamellar thickness. With lamellar straightening up to 80 mmHg, fibrils become oriented and there is no further change at or above 100 mmHg. Above 80 mmHg pressures, collagen bundles are less distinct and bands, wisps, and bundles are less numerous. At 100 and 150 mmHg, collagen fibers are seen by electron microscopy to be arranged circumferentially. These fibers are abundant in the adventitia and they are arranged in bundles. The relatively few adventitial elastin fibers and short, thick elastin lamellae are not as wavy as those of the media at high pressures. Orientation of smooth muscle in the media follows that of interlamellar elastin (21).

With increasing luminal pressures (over physiologic range) the circumferential stress gradually increases but there is further increment in diameter (21). One may rightly speculate that if the increase of pressure is spread over a prolonged time period, then this gradual diameter increase is even more prominent. Such increase in diameter of the aortic wall will not only increase wall stress due to the increase in radius, but it will predispose for aortic wall-tear by another mechanism as well, i.e., by necessarily thinning the aortic wall as a result of the enlargement.

As the aorta continues to dilate the geometry of the aortic segment changes its shape from cylindrical to ellipsoidal to spherical. This change in the geometry affects the wall stress as follows. The longitudinal stress increases with the dilation, i.e.,

$$S_l = \frac{PR'}{2T},$$

where R' is a new radius of the dilated aortic segment. The circumferential stress, on the other hand, does not increase in a simple manner but has a value between

$$\frac{PR'}{T}$$

(for a cylindrical shape) and

$$\frac{PR'}{2T}$$

(for a spherical shape). Thus, for an ellipsoidal geometry of dilated segment S_c is between

$$\frac{PR'}{T} \text{ and } \frac{PR'}{2T}.$$

In other words, the circumferential stress tends to increase by virtue of the increase in the radius but tends to decrease by virtue of the change in the shape of the aorta. The net result may be that it does not change much with the dilation. Both the longitudinal and the circumferential stresses are further modified by thinning of the aortic wall. Overall, as the aorta dilates the longitudinal stress increases faster and by a larger amount, whereas circumferential stress increases slower and by a smaller amount. The tear in the aorta could then be produced by either longitudinal or circumferential stress. Furthermore, both of these stresses are highest on the inner surface of the aorta and they decrease through the media towards the adventitia. Consequently, the circumferential or longitudinal wall stress overwhelms the strength of the inner layer (S_c or $S_l > W_{sti}$) but not that of the outer layer (S_c or $S_l < W_{sto}$) – thus, the inner layer tears but the outer one does not, and dissection develops.

Considering all this, how can we *prevent dissection in Marfan patients?*

Blood-pressure-lowering regimens in Marfan syndrome are ineffective for the simple reason that the great majority of patients has blood pressure levels within physiological limits and they would not tolerate well a further decrease. Thus, *management of aortic enlargement must be the key* to preventing dissection because enlargement of the aorta, which inevitably occurs in the "pre-dissection phase", is an anatomical feature which makes the situation uniquely manageable by surgical means. The surgical significance of a aortic diameter as the main determinate of wall stress is reflected in the work of Williams, who successfully treated a limited number of patients with chronic aortic dissection by removing the dissected inner layer of the aneurysm and reducing the diameter of the remaining wall formed by the outer layer of the dissection. Of his 13 patients operated with this method over a 12-year period, eleven are alive and well, with the observation period ranging from 1 month to 12 years (20).

We believe, however, that to operate on patients with Marfan syndrome after aortic dissection has already developed is often to late. Not only is the morbidity and mortality associated with such operations very high but also, in most cases, only the area of intimal tear and surrounding dissection is controlled while the pathological process, which often extends past the aortic arch and into the descending aorta or lower, is not addressed and remains untreated, raising the high probability of complications later in patient's life. Evidently, we should operate on Marfan patients before dissection occurs.

Radical surgical methods consisting of ascending aortic resection and replacement have been reported (4, 6). These procedures, however, are complicated and have relatively high mortality rates related to hemorrhage, dissection, residual aortic regurgitation, leaking prostheses, and recurrent aneurysm formation. Naturally, this also brings up the question of whether, and if yes, when should such a tremendous undertaking occur in a young, asymptomatic person who has only moderate dilatation of the ascending aorta? This dilemma was expressed eloquently in an editorial by Tom Treasure:

> *Because a patient with Marfan syndrome who has acute dissection faces almost certain death, there may be no alternative but emergency surgery with its high operative mortality. Dissection is the cause of sudden death in most patients with Marfan syndrome. So, the logical approach would be to operate electively before dissection occurs. If we were confident that the surgical risks were small, we would have little difficulty making such a recommendation. But in a young, symptom-free*

patient leading an active life, working full time, and caring for a family, we must feel justified in taking even a moderate surgical risk. If there is significant aortic valve regurgitation, surgery may be indicated on more established grounds – to relieve symptoms or to preserve deteriorating left ventricular function. This makes the decision easier, but in a patient who is entirely symptom-free the prospect of aortic root replacement may seem daunting. This is the dilemma we face in deciding when to recommend elective aortic root replacement in symptom-free patients with Marfan syndrome (19).

The solution to this dilemma is to design a procedure which fulfills the criteria of aortic wall stabilization with minimal operative risk. Such a procedure would be based on understanding the hemodynamics of the disease, which has two primary components, abnormally high aortic wall stress and inherent weakness of the aortic wall. The former is caused by an increase in diameter, the latter by structural weakness enhanced by wall thinness due to the dilatation. Also, in order to justify the operation's application in a special group of young individuals with often asymptomatic ascending aortic dilatation, it should have low morbidity and mortality.

The procedure we propose indeed fulfills the criteria by decreasing the aortic diameter by aortoplasty and then reinforcing the aortic wall by encasing the aorta in a well-tailored Dacron vascular prosthesis.

Method

The ascending aortic aneurysm and the heart are exposed through the usual midline sternotomy incision. The pericardium is opened and the ascending aorta is separated from the main pulmonary artery. If the aneurysm involves the origin of the innominate artery, the surgical dissection is carried up into the midaortic arch; usually this is not necessary. The patient is then placed on cardiopulmonary bypass with the caval vein cannulated transatrially and the arterial return accomplished through one of the femoral arteries. The left ventricle is vented through the confluence of the right pulmonary veins (Fig. 3A). The aorta is then cross-clamped distal to the aneurysm and the aortic valve is exposed through a longitudinal aortotomy which is carried into the non-coronary sinus. Myocardial protection is achieved by direct infusion of cold cardioplegic solution into the exposed coronary orifices. The aortic valve is excised and replaced with a prosthesis of the surgeon's choice (Fig. 3B). All sutures attaching the prosthesis to the aortic annulus are placed in the usual way except for the three commissural stitches. These three "anchoring sutures" are carried from the prosthesis through the aortic wall inside-out to the exterior of the aorta, tied over Teflon felt pledgets, and with the needles uncut, left to dangle. The aortotomy incision is now extended to the upper end of the aneurysmatic dilatation, and with the aortotomy incision as axis, an oval portion of the anterior aortic wall of appropriate length and size is removed, to bring the diameter of the ascending aorta down to normal (Fig. 3C). The aortotomy is now closed with running 4-0 polypropylene mattress sutures, then reinforced by a continuous "over and over" suture. Air is carefully evacuated from the interior of the heart and the aorta, and the patient is taken off cardiopulmonary bypass. A large caliber Dacron vascular graft is now measured to appropriate length, slit open longitudinally, and placed around the ascending aorta. The diameter of the graft is tailored to fit snugly but not constrict (Fig. 3D). The graft is closed anteriorly with a longi-

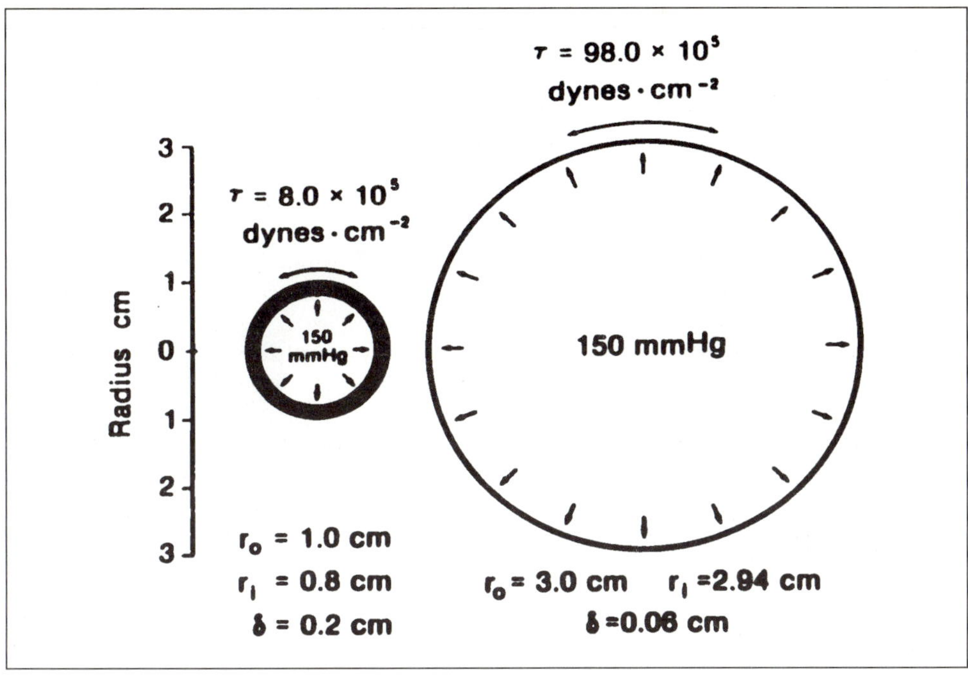

Fig. 1. End-on view of a cylinder 2 cm in diameter before and after expansion to a diameter of 6 cm. Wall area remains the same in the two figures, but wall stess ($\tau = S_c$) is greatly increased owing both to the decrease in wall thickness ($T = \delta$) and to the increase in inside radius (ri = R). From: Sumner DS (1989) Essential hemodynamic principles. (In: Rutherford R (ed), Vascular Surgery. W B Saunders Company, Philadelphia, pp 18–41. Reprinted with permission).

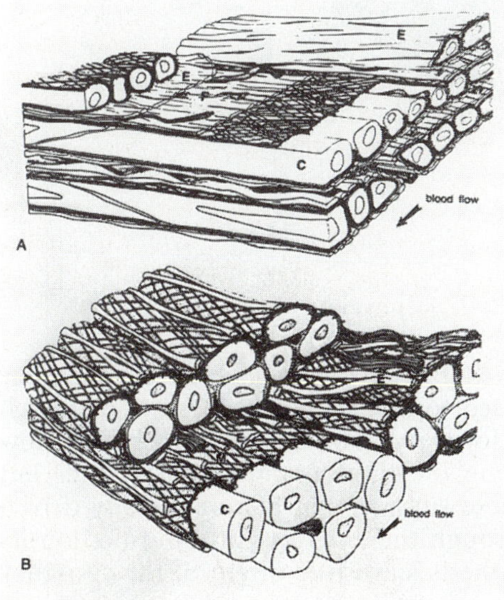

Fig. 2. Schematic representation of the lamellar organization of elastic *(A)* and muscular *(B)* arteries. The transverse (circumferential) plane of section is indicated by *C* and the longitudinal axis by *L*. Each unit is composed of a group of commonly oriented smooth muscle cells *(Ce)* surrounded by matrix *(M)* consiting of basal lamina and a fine meshwork of collagen and surrounded by elastic fibers *(E)* oriented in the same direction as the long axes of the cells. Wavy collagen bundles *(F)* lie between the elastic fibers. The elastic lamellae are much better defined in the elastic arteries *(A)* than in the muscular arteries *(B)*. (From: Clark JM, Glagov S: Transmural organization of the arterial media: The lamellar unit revisited. Arteriosclerosis 5: 19–34, 1985. By permission of the American Heart Association, Inc.)

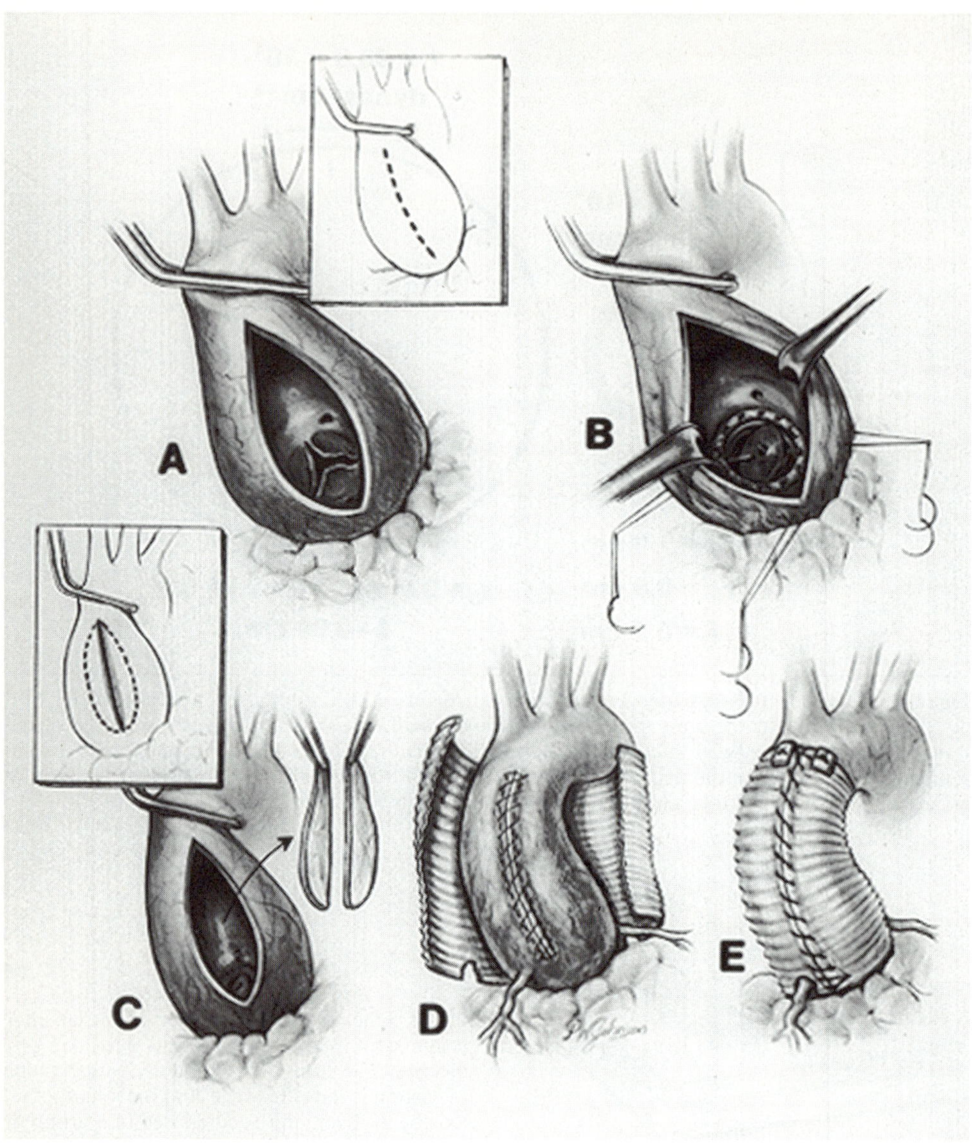

Fig. 3. Steps of the operative procedure (see text).

tudinal 2-0 polypropylene running suture. At the proximal edge of the vascular graft, small semicircular pieces may be excised to assure that it does not encroach on the origin of the coronary arteries. The lower edge of the Dacron graft is now anchored to the prosthetic aortic valve using the three commissural sutures left "dangling" on the outside of the aorta. These sutures, which were already driven through the aortic wall, are now carried through the Dacron graft and tied on its outside. Again, care is exerted that the prosthesis leaves the origin of the coronary arteries free (Fig. 3E).

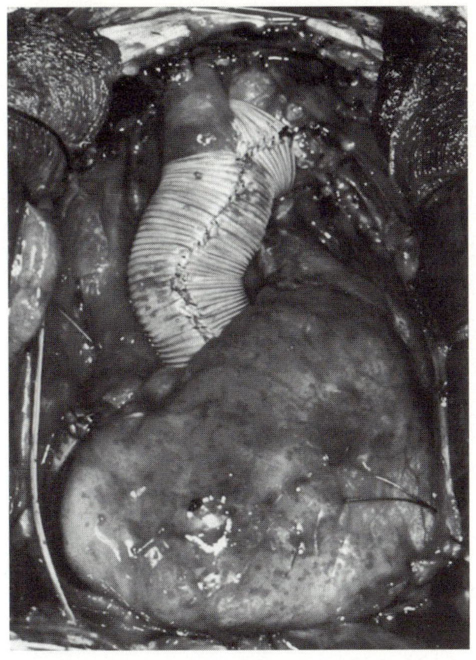

Fig. 4. The operative site following aortoplasty and external reinforcement of the proximal aortic arch.

This procedure takes about 2 hours to perform and usually requires no more than 45 minutes on cardiopulmonary bypass. Because of the single linear aortic closure, bleeding and hemorrhagic complications are extremely rare and the surgical trauma certainly does not exceed that of an "uncomplicated" aortic valve replacement.

Eighteen such operations have been performed on our service, with the follow-up period ranging from 1 to 16 years. Fourteen of these operations involved aortoplasty and aortic valve replacement, four involved external wall reinforcement only (two of the ascending aorta only and the other two of the entire aortic arch). No technical difficulties were encountered in the course of the surgery. There was no operative mortality. We know of no postoperative rupture.

Conclusions and Summary

Anatomical and blood-pressure-related factors which may cause aortic dissection with special attention to aortic dilatation are discussed. While pharmacological means to decrease wall stress are undoubtedly the appropriate approach to minimize the chance of dissection in hypertensive patients, in Marfan syndrome, if the aortic enlargement is significant, preferential consideration should be given to handling the situation by aortoplasty and external wall reinforcement, and aortic valve replacement if necessary. Aortoplasty should be dedicated to restore the aortic lumen down to a normal diameter and it should be applied only if dissection has not yet occurred or if the aneurysm is not extremely large and irregular. In such cases resection and ascending aorta replacement should be performed.

References

1. Baer RW, Taussig HB, Oppenheimer EH (1943) Congenital aneurysmal dilatation of the aorta associated with arachnodactyly. Johns Hopkins Med J 72: 309–331
2. Bergel DH (1961) The dynamic elastic properties of the arterial wall. J Physiol 156: 445–469
3. Clark JM, Glagov S (1985): Transmural organization of the arterial media: The lamellar unit revisited. Arteriosclerosis 5: 19–34
4. Crawford ES (1983) Marfan's syndrome: Broad spectral surgical treatment of cardiovascular manifestations. Ann Surg 198: 487–505
5. Etter LE, Glover LP (1943) Arachnodactyly complicated by dislocated lens and death from rupture of dissecting aneurysm of aorta. JAMA 123: 88–89
6. Gott VL, Pyeritz RE, Magovern GJ Jr, Cameron DE, McKusick VA (1986) Surgical treatment of aneurysm of the ascending aorta in the Marfan syndrome: Results of composite-graft repair in 50 patients. N Engl J Med 314: 1070–1074
7. Hallock P, Benson IC (1937) Studies on the elastic properties of human isolated aorta. J Clin Invest 16: 595–602
8. Hirata K, Triposkiadis F, Sparks E, Bowen J, Wooley CF, Boudoulas H (1991) The Marfan syndrome: Abnormal aortic elastic properties. J Amer Coll Card 18: 57–63
9. Marfan AB (1896) Un cas de deformation congenitale des quatres membres, plus prononcee aux extremites, caracterisee par l'allongement des os avec un certain degre d'amincussement. Bull Soc Chir Paris 13: 220–225
10. McDonald GR, Schaff HV, Pyeritz RE, McKusick VA, Gott VL (1981) Surgical management of patients with the Marfan syndrome and dilatation of the ascending aorta. J Thorac Cardiovasc Surg 81: 180–186
11. Murdoch JL, Walker BA, Halpern BL, Kuzma JW, McKusick VA (1972) Life expectancy and causes of death in the Marfan syndrome. N Engl J Med 286: 804–808
12. Pyeritz RE, McKusick VA (1979) The Marfan syndrome diagnosis and management. N Engl J Med 300: 772–777
13. Pyeritz RE, Reider R, Fortuin NJ (1981) Aortic complications in adult Marfan syndrome are associated with the aortic root diameter (abstract). Clin Res 29: 315A
14. Reuterwall OP (1921) Über die Elastikitat der Geftisswande und die Methode Hoer noheren Priefung. Acta Med Scand, suppl. 2: 1–175
15. Roberts WC (1981) Aortic dissection: Anatomy, consequences and causes. Am Heart J 101: 195–214
16. Sisk HE, Sahka KG, Pyeritz RE (1985) The Marfan syndrome in early childhood: Analysis of 15 patients diagnosed less than 4 years of age. Am J Cardiol 52: 353–358
17. Stromberg DD, Weiderheilm CA (1969) Viscoelastic description of a collagenous tissue in simple elongation. J Appl Physiol 26: 857
18. Summer DS (1989) Esential hemodynamic principles. In: Rutherford, R (ed) Vascular Surgery. WB Saunders Company, Philadelphia, pp 18–41
19. Treasure Thomas (1993) Elective replacement of the aortic root the Marfan's syndrome. Br Heart J 69: 101–103
20. Williams GM (1993) Treatment of chronic expanding dissecting aneurysms of the descending thoracic and operative abdominal aorta by extended aortotomy, removal of the dissected intima enclosure. J Vasc Surgery (in press)
21. Wolinsky H, Glagov S (1964) Structural basis for the static mechanical properties of the aortic media. Circ Res 14: 400–413
22. Yin FCP, Brin KP, Ting C-T, Pyeritz RE (1989) Arterial hemodynamic indexes in Marfan's syndrome. Circulation 79: 854–862

Authors' adress:
Francis Robicsek, MD
The Sanger Clinic, PA
1001 Blythe Blvd, Suite 300
Charlotte, NC 28203 USA

Management of aortic valve incompetence in patients with Marfan syndrome

M. H. Yacoub*, T. M. Sundt, N. Rasmi

Harefield Hospital*, Harefield and Royal Brompton & National Heart Hospitals, Sydney Street, London, England

Introduction

Follwoing the original description of the skeletal manifestation of Marfan syndrome (1, 2), a relatively long time elapsed before recognition of the potentially lethal cardiovascular manifestations of the disease (3–5), and only recently has it become evident that these are the main determinants of prognosis of affected individuals (6). If uncorrected, these manifestations can lead to severe disability or death at a young age. Although prolapse of the mitral valve is the most common cardiovascular manifestation of the condition, pathology of the ascending aorta and root is frequently seen and is the most common manifestation requiring surgical intervention. Aortic regurgitation may result from aneurysmal dilitation or dissection. The purpose of this chapter is to describe the management of aortic regurgitation in Marfan syndrome with particular reference to the use of a valve-conserving operation combined with radical excision of the sinuses, a technique introduced by us 15 years ago, and the place of prophylactic surgical treatment which, in our view, is closely linked to valve repair.

Plan of management

To formulate a rational plan of management it is essential to define the pathophysiology of aortic regurgitation in Marfan syndrome, its natural history, and relation to secondary changes in the aortic valve and left ventricle as well as dissection. This should be coupled with knowledge of the long-term results of treatment (medical, surgical or combined) in terms of survival, quality of life and incidence of complications. Data relating to some of these areas are still incomplete and require further research and the use of predictions to supplement the known facts.

Pathophysiology and natural history of aortic regurgitation in Marfan

Definition of pathophysiology depends on thorough understanding of the functional anatomy of the aortic valve complex. This comprises the sinuses of Valsalva, the surgical anulus, valve cusps and commissures. Each of these components plays an essential role in maintaining "normal" aortic valve function. The aortic sinuses maintain the three-dimensional shape of the aortic valve complex, create vortices which ensure smooth opening and closure of the cusps, and through their mobility during the different parts of the cardiac cycle reduce the mechanical stress on the valve cusps. These functions are dependent on the shape and structure of the sinuses which have a well defined elastic media continuous with the media of the ascending aorta and firmly attached to the fibrous aortic anulus (Fig. 1). The latter is a crown-shaped "ring" which is continuous, with the right and left fibrous trigones at the mid points of the non- and left aortic sinuses, respectively. Although the anulus is a continuous structure all around the aortic orifice, it is slightly less well defined in the region of the right coronary sinus. The anulus is a firm triangular (in cross-section) fibrous structure which serves as an anchor to the aortic media and the bases of the cusps (Fig. 1) while maintaining mobility of the aortic valve complex in a three-dimensional plane. Thus the structure of the anulus suits perfectly its functions. The aortic cusps consist of three functional units: the region next to the anulus which acts as a hinge, a body and a coapting surface. The sophisticated function of the cusps depends on their shape coupled to the specific

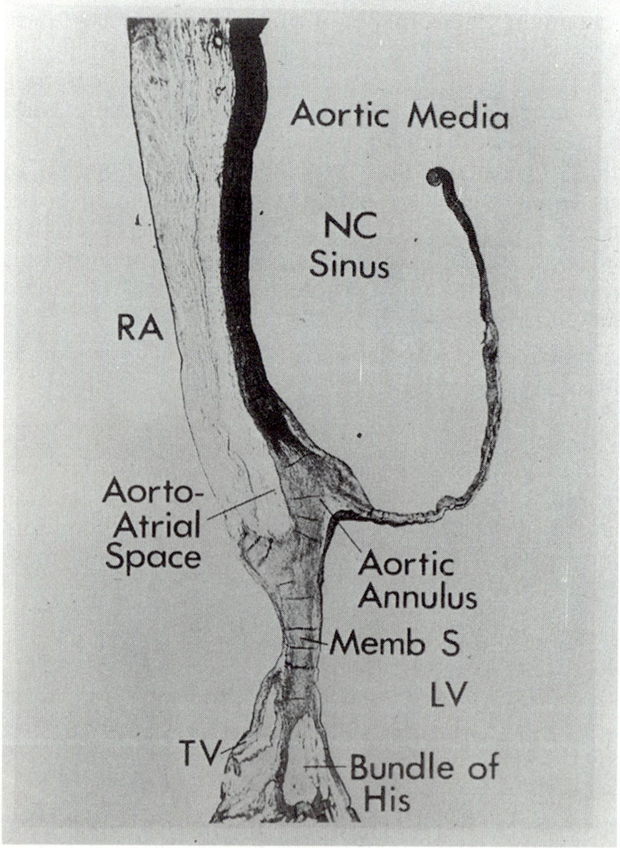

Fig. 1: Photomicrograph of a longitudinal section through the region at the anterior half of the noncoronary cusp (elastic stain) shaving the relations of the aorto-atrial space, the aortic media, and the aortic annulus.

viscoelastic properties which are a function of the thickness and tissue composition of each component of the cusp. The cusp leaflet is formed of a fibrous core, termed the fibrosa, covered on either side by the ventricularis and spongiosa which are lined by endothelial cells.

The commissures act as fibrous pillars to suspend the valve cusps, particularly the free edges which play an important part in cusp coaptation. The commissures themselves are dependent on the aortic sinuses and the sinotubular junction for support and maintenance of the appropriate geometry.

We believe that aortic regurgitation in Marfan syndrome is, at least initially, due to abnormalities of the aortic sinuses and sinotubular junction although secondary changes in the valve leaflets ultimately occur. Progressive dilatation of the aorta results in obliteration of the sinotubular junction with progressive involvement of the sinuses. This results in wide separation of the commissures in relation to each other and failure of coaptation of the cusps. The turbulence resulting from aortic regurgitation produces progressive fibrosis and retraction, initially of the coapting surfaces, and later the body of the cusps, which can make the valve unsuitable for repair. We therefore believe that the changes in the leaflets themselves are secondary and are potentially preventable by "early" repair. We further believe that the term

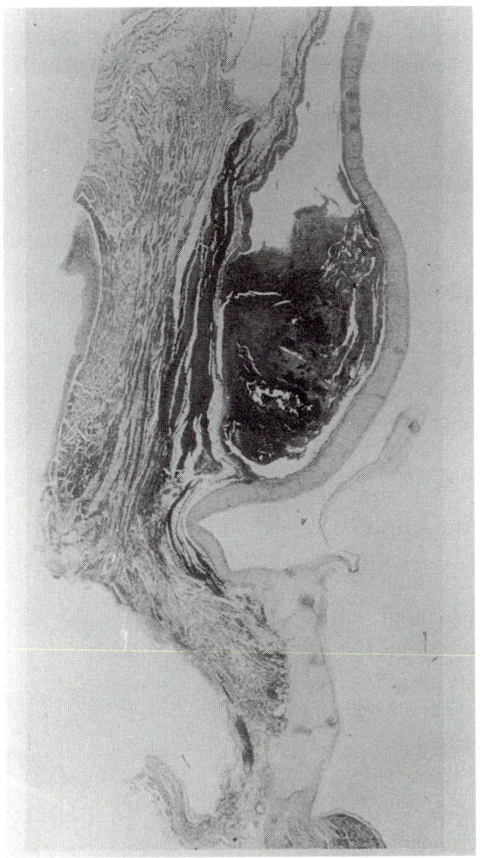

Fig. 2: Photomicrograph of a longitudinal section of the aortic root through the region of the non-coronary cusp from a patient with an acute dissection (hematoxylin and eosin stain). Note that the dissection extends to, but not beyond, the aortic annulus.

anulo-aortic ectasia, frequently used to describe the aortic root in Marfan syndrome, is misleading as it implies primary abnormality of the aortic anulus which we believe not to be the case.

The exact rate of dilatation of the sinotubular junction and sinuses appears to be variable and could be influenced by several factors which include the exact mutation in the fibrillin gene, the characteristics of the blood pressure which acts as the distending force and the size of the sinuses themselves which determines wall tension by the Law of LaPlace.

Relation of aortic regurgitation to dissection

Aortic dissection, which is common in Marfan syndrome, is usually due to an intimal tear in the proximal ascending aorta with the dissection involving the sinotubular junction and aortic sinuses with resulting prolapse of one or more the commissures. This produces or increases the severity of aortic regurgitation. The dissection, however, never crosses or involves the anulus or cusps (Fig. 2). This observation renders our reparative procedure (see later), which involves excision of the sinuses, ideal for these patients unless there are pre-existing severe secondary changes involving the valve cusps.

In some patients with strong family history of dissection at a young age, acute dissection with catastrophic aortic regurgitation or rupture can be the first cardiovascular manifestation. Identification of these patients is important as prophylactic surgical treatment could be considered.

Left ventricular function in Marfan aortic regurgitation

Although varying degrees of left ventricular dysfunction have been described in patients with Marfan syndrome, left ventricular function is usually adequate in patients with mild to moderate regurgitation. Severe irreversible left ventricular dysfunction secondary to aortic regurgitation occurs later than secondary changes in the aortic valve cusps. This is another factor in favour of operating relatively early on these patients.

Medical treatment

This is usually designed to reduce the distending pressure, as well as its rate of rise, using pharmacologic means. This may delay the onset of regurgitation and possibly reduce the incidence of dissection (7).

Once left ventricular dysfunction is established, antifailure treatment could also be of value. Although important, medical treatment is limited in scope and is commonly combined with surgical therapy.

Surgical options

The ideal operation for Marfan aortic regurgitation should eliminate all abnormal tissue, thereby preventing or minimising the risk of aneurysmal recurrence or rupture, should allow for growth given the young age at which surgical intervention may be required, and obviate the necessity of the use of anticoagulants – with their known risks and inconveniences. In addition, such an operation should be free from the risk of late endocarditis or valve degeneration; the search for this ideal operation continues. We believe that an essential component of any operation to be used is radical excision of the aortic sinuses. Currently this can be achieved by

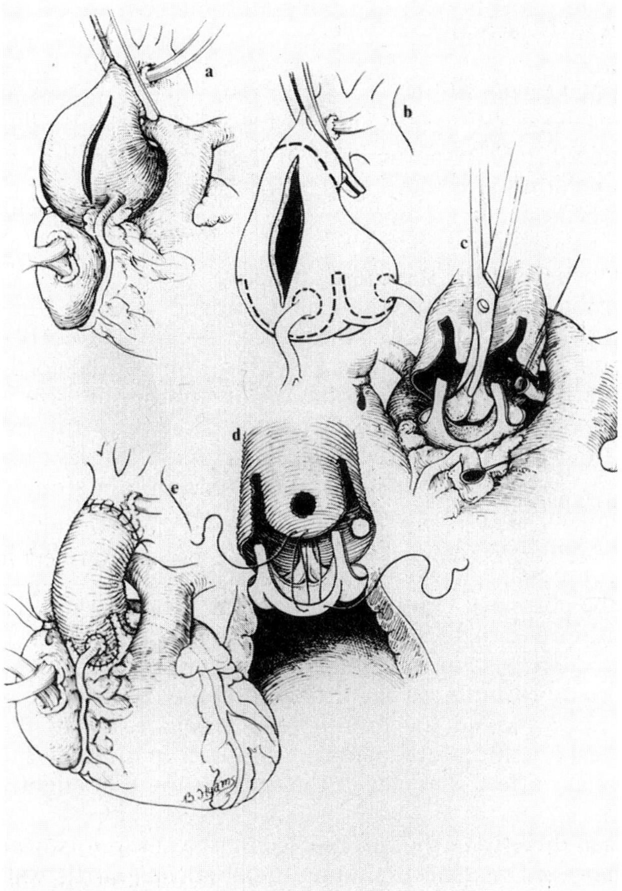

Fig. 3: Technique of radical excision of the aortic root presserving the native aortic valve. a) After establishing cardiopulmonary bypass with inflow via the proximal arch or the common femoral artery, a crossclamp is applied and the aneurysm opened using a standard ventricle aortotomy into the non coronary sinus. b) and c) The wall at the ascending aorta and root is radically excised to within 1 mm at the surgical anulus of the aortic valve, and leaving small buttons around the coronary ostia. d) An appropriately tailored dacron tube graft is then sewn to the aortic anulus and the coronary buttons reimplanted. e) The reconstructed root.

a variety of techniques. The first successful approach to achieve this was that described by Bentall and DeBono in 1968, who described composite aortic root and valve replacement using a prosthetic valve and a dacron graft with reimplantation of the coronary ostia (8). This remains the most commonly applied operation and has many advantages which include the standard nature (familiarity) and low risk of the procedure, as well as the perceived long-term durability (9). The disadvantages of this procedure, however, include all the known complications of prosthetic aortic valves (10) and the possibility of excising a potentially functional aortic valve. The use of a free standing aortic homograft originally introduced by us in 1976 (11), has not been widely used in patients with Marfan syndrome because of the misconception that the aortic anulus is abnormal and therefore liable to dilate and produce homograft regurgitation.

This technique can be used in Marfan syndrome and has all the advantages of homografts (12), but suffers from the lack of availability of homografts and, more importantly, the relatively limited durability particularly in the younger age groups (12). However, the risk of re-operation after homograft root replacement (13) has been shown to be low and the necessity for re-operation decreases with advancing age (12).

The third option, which we believe to be the most attractive, is a technique of radical excision of the aortic root, with resuspension of the aortic valve and implantation of the coronary ostia (Fig. 3) which was introduced by us in 1979 (14). The technique consists of excision of the aortic sinuses to within 1 mm of the aortic anulus, which is a well defined structure. A dacron tube of the appropriate size is fashioned to have three tongue-shaped processes to match the three reconstituted sinuses. The size and shape of the new dacron sinuses is determined by elevating the three mobilised commissures and holding them up under tension in a straight upwards direction (Fig. 3). Myocardial protection is achieved by cold crystalloid or blood cardioplegia. The dacron sinuses are then sutured to the aortic anulus which acts as an excellent suturing material even in patients with acute dissection of the aortic sinuses. Finally, the coronary "buttons" are prepared by excising the surrounding aortic wall to within 1 mm of the orifice; the conus artery, which commonly arises by a separate orifice next to the right coronary orifice, is included in the button. No attempt is made to mobilise the proximal coronary arteries as the ostia are often displaced upwards and the buttons can always reach to the dacron tube without tension. Two orifices are made in the dacron tube at the appropriate point for each coronary artery. The size of the orifice should be slightly smaller than that of the button.

The latter is then anastomosed directly to the orifice placing the sutures as near as possible to the actual coronary orifice, thus excluding the abnormal aortic wall from the circulation.

Timing of operation and the concept of prophylaxis

Most patients with Marfan syndrome will develop aortic regurgitation either acutely or progressively with secondary changes in the valve cusps and left ventricle. The plan of management should aim at preventing symptoms, risk of rupture and secondary irreversible structural changes. This can be achieved by combining medical and surgical treatment through anticipating irreversible changes and offering operation before their onset. Family history and regular monitoring of the size of the aortic root and the state of the aortic valve and left ventricle by non invasive means can act as predictors to help the decision process. It is hoped that evolution of molecular markers of rapid progression could be of additional help. If such a programme is evolved and adhered to, the valve conserving operation described here should be applicable to the majority of patients requiring operation with a greater likelihood of long term success. In our experience, due to late referral, valve conserving operations were achieved in only approximately 50% of patients. It is hoped that this will be remedied in the future.

Results

During the last 20 years, we have operated on 232 patients with aneurysms of the ascending aorta and root at the Harefield, Royal Brompton and National Heart Hospitals. In this series, approximately one-third (74 patients) satisfied the clinical criteria of Marfan syndrome. The indication for operation in the Marfan group was chronic dessection in 17 (23%); acute dissection in 16 (22%) and chronic aneurysm in 41 (54%).

The age distribution in the three groups is shown in Fig. 4. There was a high peak incidence of acute dissection amongst patients in their 20s while the age distribution for isolated aneurysms or chronic dissection was bell-shaped. Root repair was performed in 36 patients (50%) including 7 patients who had cusp extension with human dura mater or calf pericardium. The remaining 38 patients underwent composite root and valve replacement with a variety of valve substitutes including homografts in 24, Starr-Edwards ball valves in 13 and a Hancock xenograft in 1.

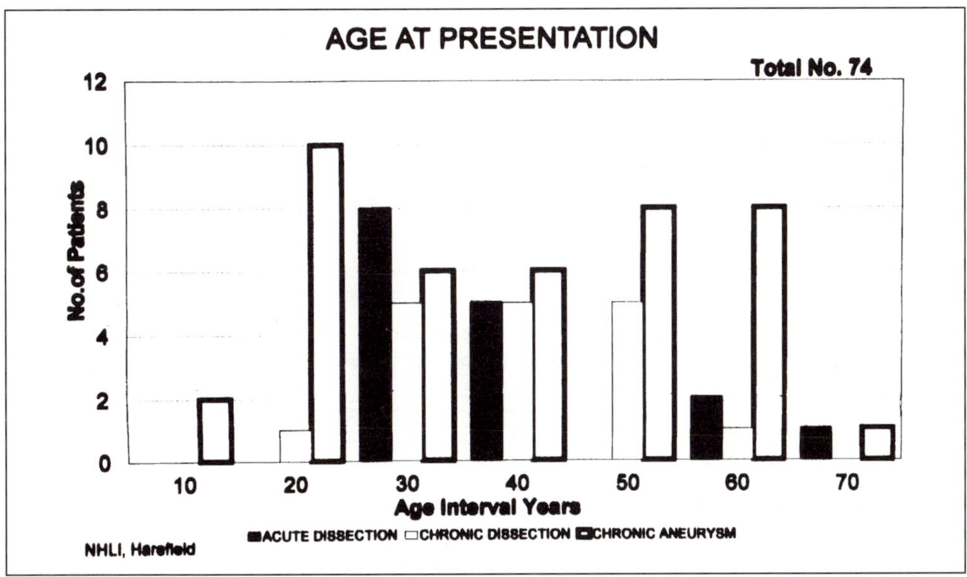

Fig. 4: Age distribution of patients with the Marfan syndrome undergoing operative procedures on the aortic root separated by indication for intervention.

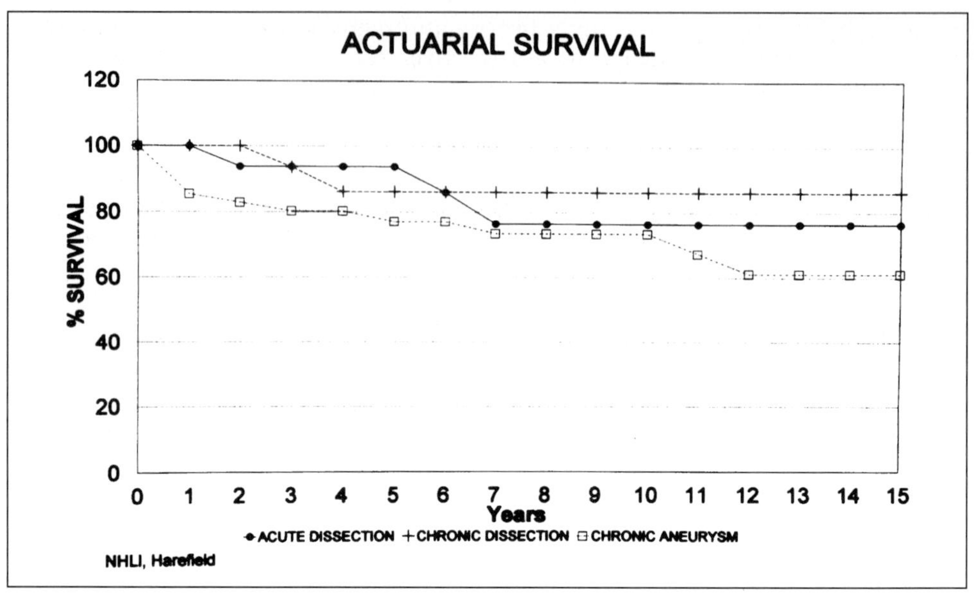

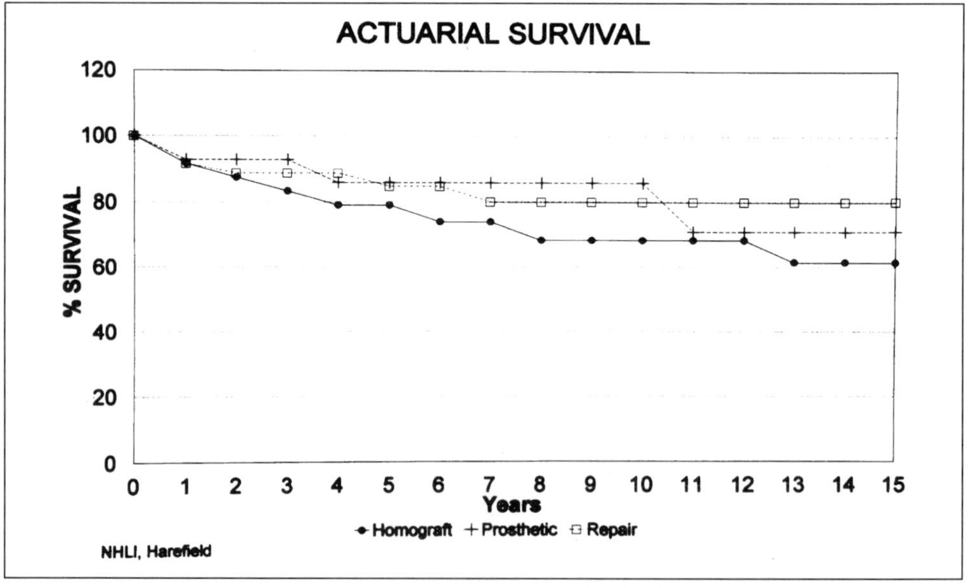

Fig. 5: Acutuarial survival following surgery of the aortic root. a) Survival by indication for intervention. b) Survival by procedure.

The overall 30-day mortality throughout the 20-year period was 8.1% (Table 1), falling to approximately one-half that during the last 5 years. There were no early deaths in the 33 patients presenting with acute or chronic dissection aneurysms. The causes of early deaths are shown in Table 2. Most of the deaths occurred in patients with severe left ventricular dysfunction, which could have possibly been avoided by earlier referral.

During the period of follow-up, which ranged from 3 months to 20 years (mean 5–7 years), 13 patients died, representing a late mortality of 17.6%. The actuarial

Table 1: Early and late mortality

		Early Mortality#	Late Mortality*	Total
By presentation:	(n =)			
Acute dissection	(16)	0	4 (25%)	4 (25%)
Chronic dissection	(17)	0	6 (35%)	6 (35%)
Chronic aneurysm	(41)	6 (14.6%)	3 (7.4%)	9 (22%)
By procedure:				
Homograft	(24)	2 (8.3%)	7 (29%)	9 (37.5%)
Prosthetic	(14)	1 (7.1%)	2 (14%)	3 (21%)
Repair	(36)	3 (8.3%)	4 (11%)	7 (19%)
Total	74	6 (8.1%)	13 (17%)	19 (26%)

Early mortality = within 30 days of operation
* Follow up 3 months to 20 years, mean = 5.7 years

Table 2: Causes of death

Early death		Late death	
Chronic aneurysm (n = 41)			
Left ventricular failure	3	Left ventricular failure	1
Arrhythmia	1	Ruptured thoraco abdominal aneurysm	3
Haemorrhage	1		
Multisystem failure	1		
Acute dissections (n = 16)			
None		Bacterial endocarditis	1
		Unknown	2
Chronic dissections (n = 17)			
None		Myocardial infarction	1
		Renal failure	1
		Intraoperative during second procedure	1
		Unknown	3

survial of patients undergoing the three types of operation is shown in Fig. 5. This shows a trend of patients undergoing valve repair to have a better survival when compared to patients undergoing composite root replacement using prosthetic valves or homograft root replacement. This, however, did not reach statistical significance.

The main cause of late death (Table 3) was aneurysms of the distal segments of the arterial system, emphasising the need for long-term follow up of these patients to diagnose and anticipate problems. Re-operation on the aortic valve was required in 9 patients (12.2%) (Table 3).

Only 3 patients in the valve repair group required re-operation, due to recurrent aortic regurgitation in two and bacterial endocarditis in one. In the homograft group, three valves failed, requiring re-operation due to degeneration and two for bacterial endocarditis. Amongst the prosthetic valve group, only one developed prosthetic valve malfunction and required re-operation. Amongst all the patients undergoing re-operation, there was one death.

Conclusions

Aortic regurgitation with or without dissection of the ascending aorta and root remains one of the most important causes of morbidity and mortality in patients with the Marfan syndrome. A management plan based on understanding of the pathophysiology of aortic regurgitation in Marfan syndrome and predicting irreversible changes is suggested. The timely use of surgical procedures aimed at wide excision of the diseased sinuses and, wherever possible, preserving the aortic valve combined with regular follow-up to detect and treat aneurysms of the peripheral vessels should improve the prognosis and quality of life of patients with the Marfan syndrome.

References

1. Marfan A-B (1896): Un cas de deformation congenitale des quatre membres plus prononcee aux extremites caracterisee par l'allongement des os avec un certain degre d'amincissement. Bull Mem Soc Med Hop Paris (ser 3) 13: 220–226
2. Marfan A-B (1938): La dolichostenomelie (dolichomelie, arachnodactylie). Ann Med 44: 5–29
3. Etter LE, Glover LP (1943): Arachnodactyly complicated by dislocated lens and death from rupture of dissecting aneurysm of aorta. J Am Med Assoc 123: 88–89
4. Baer RW, Taussig HB, Oppenheimer EH (1943): Congenital aneurysmal dilatation of the aorta associated with arachnodactyly. Bull Johns Hopkins Hosp 72: 309–331
5. McKusick VA (1955): The cardiovascular aspects of Marfan's syndrome: A heritable disorder of connective tissue. Circulation 11: 321–342
6. Murdoch JL, Walker BA, Halpern BL, Kuzma JW, McKusick VA (1972): Life expectancy and causes of death in the Marfan syndrome. N Engl J Med 286: 804–808
7. Jennifer Shores, Kenneth R Berger, Edmond A Murphy, Reed E Pyeritz (1994): Progression of aortic dilatation and the benefit of long-term B-adrenergic blockage in Marfan's Syndrome.
8. Bentall H De Bono A: A technique for complete replacement of the ascending aorta. Thorax 23: 338–339, 1968
9. Nicholas T Kouchoukos, Thomas H Wareing, suzan F Murphy, Johanna B Perrillo (1991): Sixteen-year experience with aortic root replacement. Annals of Surgery 308–320

10. Ross J Jr: Afterload mismatch in aortic and mitral valve disease: implications for surgical therapy. J Am Coll Cardiol 1985: 5: 811–826
11. Gula G, Ahmed M, Thompson R, Radley-Smith R, Yacoub M: Combined homograft replacement of the aortic valve and aortic root with reimplantation of the coronary arteries. Circulation 1976, 54: II 150.
12. Yacoub M, Rasmi N, Sundt T, Lund O, Boyland E, Radley-Smith R, Khaghani A, Mitchell A: Fourteen year experience with homovital homografts for aortic valve replacement. J Thor Cardiovasc Surg – manuscript submitted April 1994
13. Sundt TM, Rasmi N, Wong K, Radley-Smith R, Khaghani A, Yacoub M: Aortic valve reoperation following homograft root replacement: Surgical options and results. Annals of Thor Surgery – manuscript submitted July 1994.
14. Magdi Yacoub, Albert Fagan, Paolo Stassano, Rosemary Radley-Smith: Results of valve conserving operations for aortic regurgitation. Circulation 1983, 68: III, 111–321

Authors' address:
M. H. Yacoub, M. D.
Harefield Hospital
Harefield, Middx. UB9 6JH
England

Annulo-aortic ectasia – with special reference to total repair of patients with Marfan syndrome

M. V. Inberg, J. Niinikoski, V. Rantakokko, T. Savunen, E. Vänttinen

Turku University Central Hospital, Turku, Finland

During the years 1975–1993, 92 patients underwent a so-called total repair using the technique developed at our institute (3, 4). In the early 1970s, we used the supracoronary resection technique in 9 cases. Figure 1 shows the first patient ever

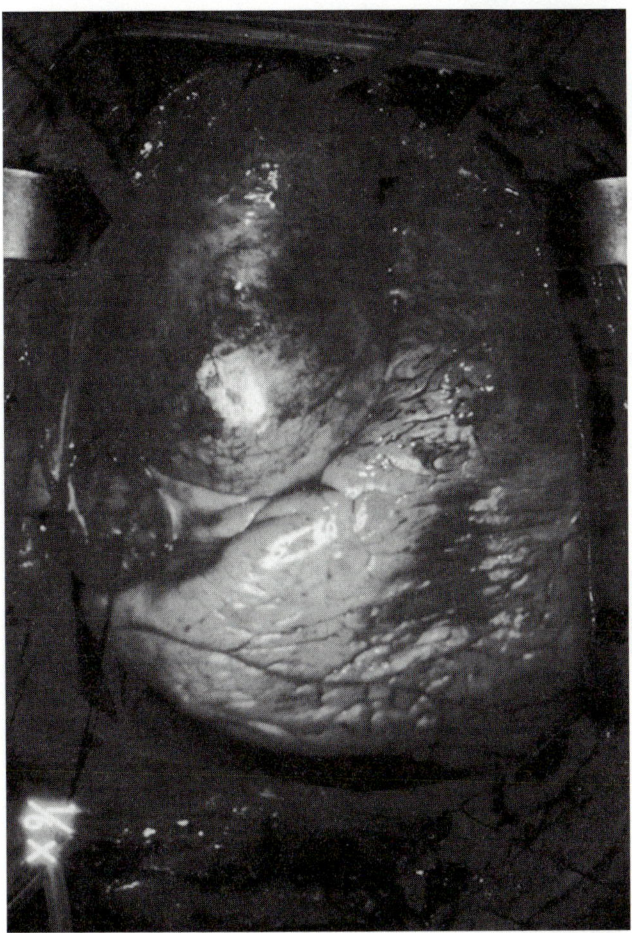

Fig. 1. Preoperative picture of a typical case of annulo-aortic ectasia. The first patient operated in Finland.

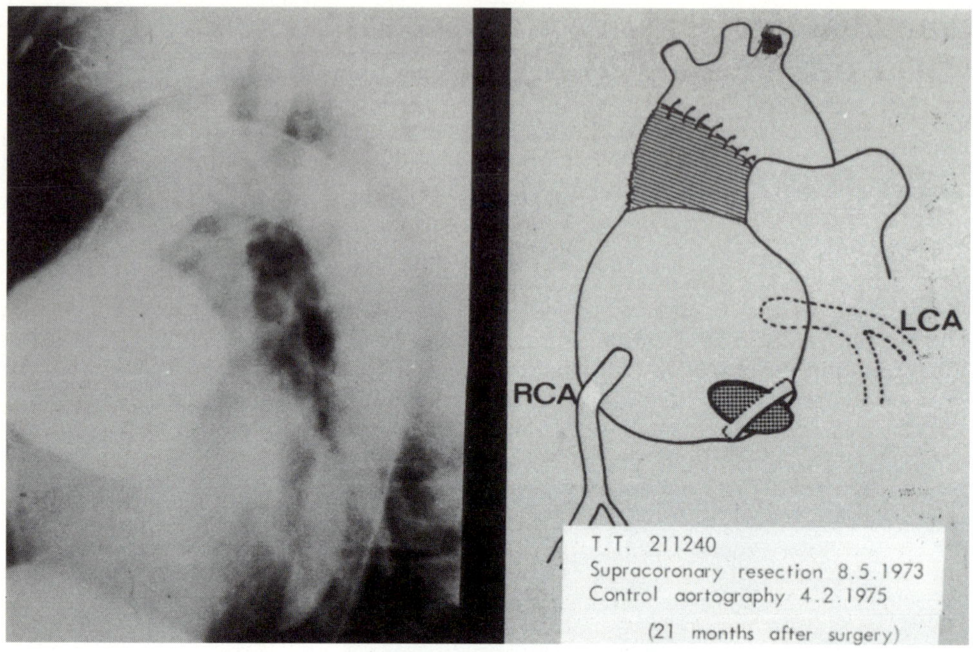

Fig. 2. Drawing and angiography of the same patient 21 months after a supracoronary resection.

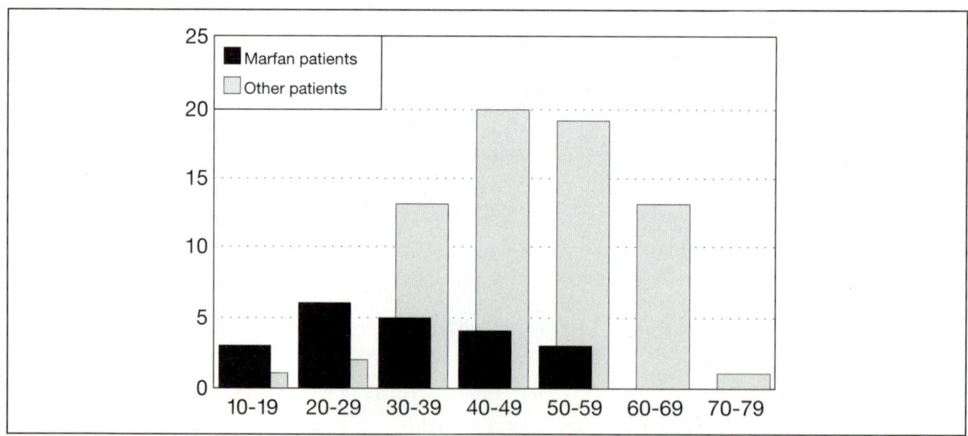

Fig. 3. Age distribution of the patients.

successfully operated in Finland. Our late results at that time were not good (2). Figure 2 shows the same patient 21 months after the operation. A huge aneurysm is evident which developed from the rim of the ascending aorta left in place above the coronary ostia. Therefore, we initiated our own technique and never used the original Bentall method (1).

Patients

This is a consecutive series. Twenty-one patients had Marfan syndrome. The Marfan patients were much younger than the others who had only a cardiovascular manifestation, annulo-aortic ectasia (Fig. 3). Three of the Marfan patients were children (5). Altogether, there were 79 elective operations. Six of these patients had chronic dissection. Emergency operations were performed in 13 cases, 11 due to acute dissection and 2 because of rupture of the aneurysm.

Surgical technique

This is a modification of the original Bentall technique. We excise the aneurysm totally (Fig. 4). The coronary origins are dissected free to avoid any tension at the anastomotic site. We have not used the commercially available composite graft, but

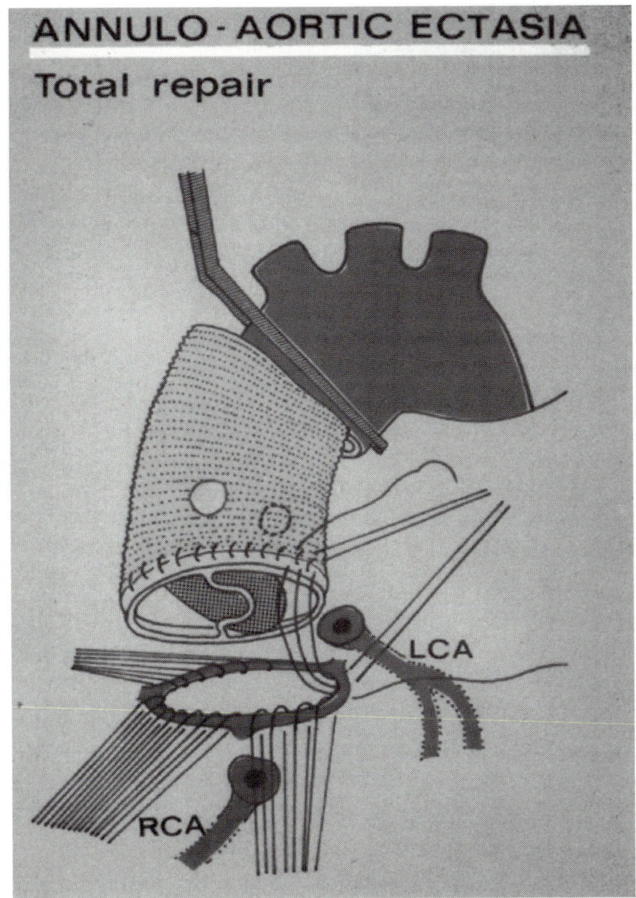

Fig. 4. The surgical technique using our total repair.

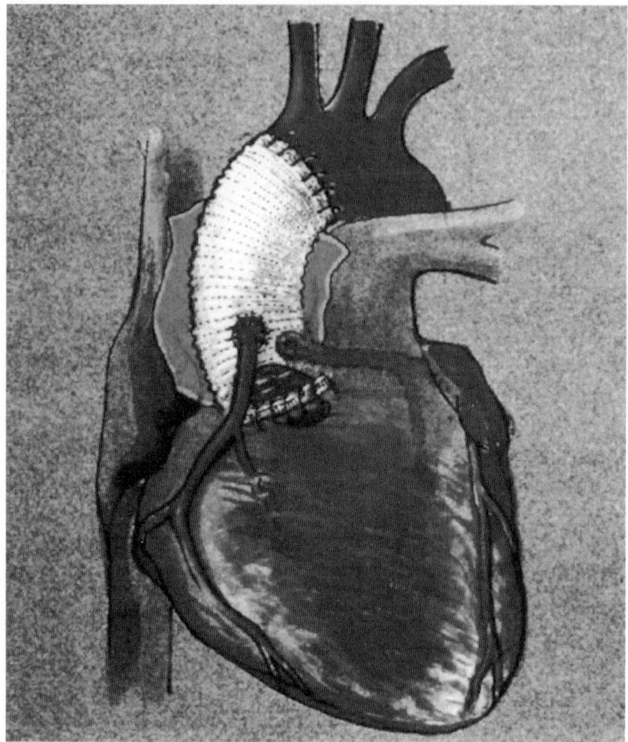

Fig. 5. Drawing showing the final result of the repair.

rather have sewn a Björk-Shiley tilting disc valve into the prosthetic tube. The final result is shown in Fig. 5. In addition to the total repair, aortic arch replacement was performed in 2 cases, coronary artery bypass-grafting in 9, and mitral valve replacement in 2 cases.

Early results

In the elective surgery group only 1 patient died (1.3%). This was the same patient shown in Fig. 2. He died following re-operation performed 6 years after the supra-coronary resection. The cause of death was myocardial infarction. In the emergency group we had 2 deaths (15.4%). Five patients required re-sternotomy because of bleeding (5.4%) and 5 developed total AV-block and needed permanent pacemaker treatment (5.4%).

Late results

Eighty-six of 92 patients were investigated by angiography 6 months after surgery. There were no pseudoaneurysms and there was a slight dilatation of the coronary

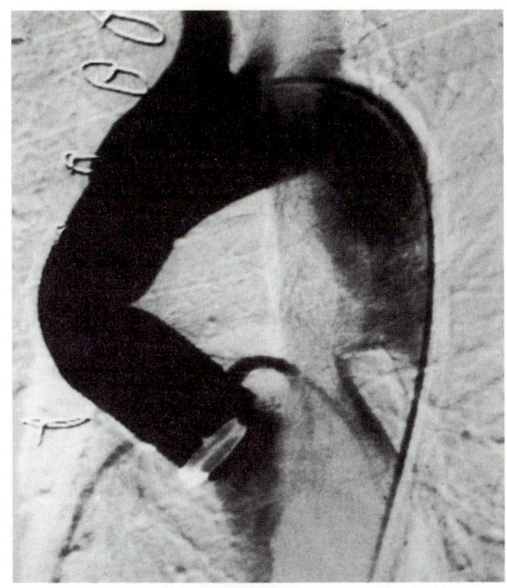

Fig. 6. Control angiography 3 years after surgery: no dilatation of the coronary origins.

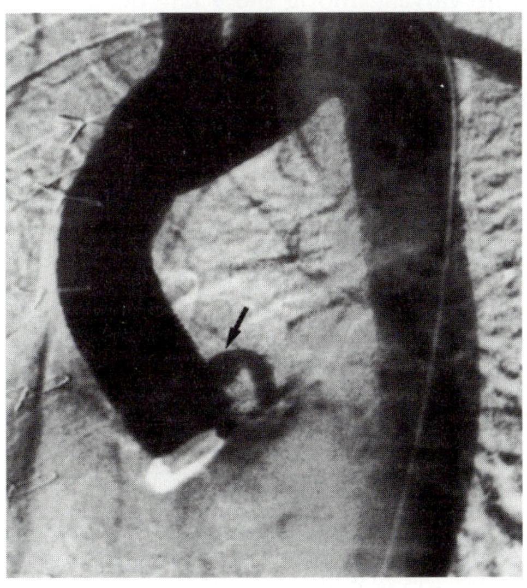

Fig. 7. Control angiography 3 years after surgery. The arrow shows the site of dilatation of the left coronary origin.

origins in only 3 patients. Three years after surgery a new angiography was made in 52 out of 71 patients. There were still no pseudoaneurysms. Slight dilatation of one or both coronary origins was seen in 15 cases. Nine of them were Marfan patients. We have not determined the clinical significance of this dilatation. Figure 6 shows a normal angiography 3 years after surgery without any ostial dilatation. Figure 7 shows a case with dilatation of the left coronary origin.

The crude survival curves are shown in Fig. 8. There was only a minor difference between the Marfan patients and the group with only annuloaortic ectasia. Three patients died due to myocardial infarction; other causes of death were rupture of the aortic arch, multiple emboli, cancer, subarachnoidal hemorrhage and suicide.

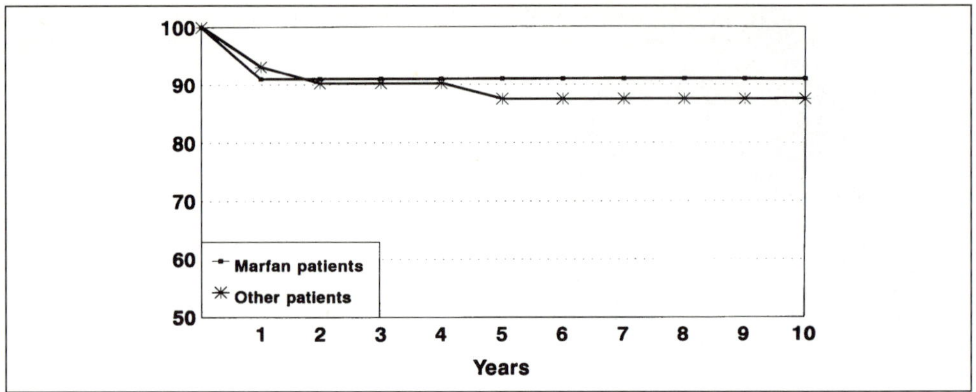

Fig. 8. The crude survival curves.

Only 2 of the 9 late deaths were valve-related. The Marfan patient who died because of emboli had stopped the use of anticoagulants. The subarachnoidal hemorrhage was due to septic emboli from the prosthetic valve. Among the 9 late deaths there were 2 Marfan patients. One died because of myocardial infarction and the other of multiple emboli. Concerning the later results, the only difference between the Marfan patients and those who had only cardiovascular manifestations was that the Marfan patients had a higher incidence of dilatation of the coronary origins. However, the significance of this dilatation is uncertain.

Conclusions

The presented series was consecutive and showed that this surgical technique is suitable for all anatomical variations. The operation is safe. The mortality and morbidity rates are fairly low. Also, the late results seem to be satisfactory. However, this method has a disadvantage in the use of a mechanical valve.

Appendix

During November 1993 – May 1994 12 additional patients were operated upon without any complications. Three of them had acute dissection.

References

1. Bentall H, DeBono A (1968) A technique for complete replacement of the ascending aorta. Thorax 23: 338–339
2. Inberg MV, Havia T, Laaksonen V, Möttönen M, Wegelius U, Vänttinen E (1977) Surgical treatment of aneurysms of the ascending aorta, with special reference to cystic medial necrosis of the aorta. Scand J Thor Cardiovasc Surg 11: 25–31
3. Inberg MV, Vänttinen E, Arola M, Wegelius U (1978) Total replacement of the ascending aorta and aortic valve with implantation of the coronary ostia in Marfan's syndrome. Scand J Thor Cardiovasc Surg 12: 15–22

4. Inberg MV; Niinikoski J, Savunen T, Vänttinen E (1985) Total repair of annulo-aortic ectasia with composite graft and reimplantation of coronary ostia: a consecutive series of 41 patients. World J Surg 9: 493–499
5. Savunen T, Niinikoski, J, Inberg MV (1984) Surgical repair of annuloaortic ectasia in children. Scand J Thor Cardiovasc Surg 18: 15–21

Authors' address:
Prof. Dr. M. V. Inberg
Department of Surgery
University of Turku
SF 20520 Turku
Finland

Marfan syndrome: The variability of operative management

J. S. Coselli, S. Büket

Baylor College of Medicine and the Methodist Hospital, Houston, Texas, USA

Introduction

Marfan syndrome is an autosomal dominant disorder of connective tissue with an incidence of approximately 1 in 20 000 (1). The disorder is characterized by clinical manifestations in the cardiovascular, ocular, and skeletal systems. As a consequence of cardiovascular complications, life expectancy is primarily reduced (2). Recent collaborative efforts have identified fibrillin as the most promising candidate gene for the Marfan syndrome (3–8). The gene coding for fibrillin has been recently localized to chromosome 15 (3, 8). The importance of this finding is that the genetic linkage of this disorder to chromosome 15 should ultimately provide DNA diagnostic analysis for patients with Marfan syndrome. Until such time when genetic diagnosis, treatment, or even prevention is available, surgical intervention will remain the mainstay of treatment for the cardiovascular manifestations that occur in greater than 95% of adults with Marfan syndrome and are responsible for the markedly reduced life expectancy of patients afflicted with the syndrome.

Patients and methods

Fifty-nine patients with Marfan syndrome were treated surgically with 66 operations upon the aorta during the 4-year period between July 18, 1989, and July 14, 1993. Included were 39 male patients (66.1%) and 20 female patients (33.9%). Their ages ranged from 21 to 63 years with a mean age of 40 years.

In addition to the cardiovascular complications, skeletal manifestations were identified in 59 patients (100%) and ocular abnormalities with Marfan syndrome in 44 (74.6%). A definitive family history of Marfan syndrome was confirmed in 39 (66.1%) patients. Twenty-two patients had four manifestations (37.3%), and 37 had three (62.7%) (9).

Thirty-six of the 59 patients (61%) had had 51 prior aortic surgical procedures. Thirty-three prior operations were for ascending aortic aneurysm and/or aortic valve replacement, 10 for descending and/or thoracoabdominal aortic replacement, 7 for ascending and/or transverse arch replacement, 1 for abdominal aortic aneurysm (Table 1). One patient had undergone prior mitral replacement for prolapse with insufficiency. There was 25 patients (42.4%) with 1 previous aortic surgery, 8 patients (13.6%) with 2 previous, 2 patients (3.4%) with 3, and 1 patient (1.7%) with 4.

Operation was carried out for dissection in 43 patients, annulo-aortic ectasia with aortic insufficiency in 12; false aneurysm of a previous composite graft in 6; fusi-

Table 1: Current and previous aortic operations

Aortic operations	Previous (n = 36)	Current (n = 59)	Total
Aortic valve	1		1
Ascending			
composite valve graft	24	17	41
false aneurysm repair	1	3	4
redo composite valve graft		3	3
ascending	7		7
Composite + arch	1	4	5
Transverse arch grafting	3	1	4
Ascending + arch	1	4	5
Ascending + arch + aortic valve	2		2
Descending	8	7	15
Thoracoabdominal	2	22	24
Descending + Thoracoabdominal		1	1
Coarctation repair		1	1
Abdominal aortic aneurysm	1	3	4
Total	51	66	117

form aneurysm in 2; coarctation, false thoracoabdominal aneurysm, and false aneurysm of a previously placed descending aortic graft in one each. Forty of the dissections were chronic (30 DeBakey Type I, 1 Type II, 9 Type III), and 3 were acute (2 Type I, 1 Type III). Of the 23 thoracoabdominal aortic aneurysms, 6 were Type I, 9 were Type II, 2 were Type III, and 6 were Type IV (based on Crawford classification) (10).

Surgical procedures were thoracoabdominal aortic aneurysm repair in 22 (33.3%), ascending aortic composite valve graft replacement in 17 (25.8%), ascending aorta and transverse arch replacement in 4 (6%), composite valve graft plus arch replacement in 4 (6%), descending thoracic aortic aneurysm repair in 7 (10.6%), ascending aortic false aneurysm repair in 3, redo composite valve graft in 3, abdominal aortic aneurysm replacement in 3, descending and thoracoabdominal aortic aneurysm replacement, transverse arch replacement and coarctation repair, one each (Table 1). Of these 59 patients, 7 were treated with a subsequent aortic operation. Of these 7, the initial operation was thoracoabdominal aortic aneurysm replacement in 5 patients. Subsequent operation in these included composite valve graft in two (2 months and 3 months), arch in 1 (12 months), distal ascending and transverse arch in 2 (3 months and 13 months). Both of the latter 2 had had prior composite graft insertion and consequently had staged total aortic replacement. One patient with composite insertion underwent coarctation repair at 2 months, and another with repair of false aneurysm repair around a composite underwent abdominal aortic aneurysm replacement at 11 months. Only one of these had had no prior aortic operation, 3 had 1, and 3 had 2 previous aortic operations.

Six patients were operated upon for complications following prior composite valve graft insertion. Three of these, who had been previously treated with composite valve graft replacement using the classical Bentall technique, presented with noninfected false aneurysm formation (11). Two of these aneurysms were treated by primary suture line repair and one by graft interposition to the right coronary artery. The remaining three patients with false aneurysm around a composite valve graft had infection (two with prior Bentall, one with prior Cabrol procedure). Each required resection and composite valve graft re-replacement for endocarditis, valve dehiscence, and false aneurysm. Each of the new grafts inserted for infection were covered with omentum as a viable pedicle.

Results

Follow-up was complete on all 59 patients (100%). In this series of patients there was 1 inhospital death for an early survival rate of 98.3% and there was 2 late deaths for a long-term survival rate of 94.9%.

A postoperative lower extremity neurologic deficit of moderate degree (paraparesis) developed in only 1 patient. This patient was a 63-year-old female operated on for ruptured thoracoabdominal aortic aneurysm. The patient was hypotensive at the initiation of the surgical procedure and underwent emergent replacement of her aorta from the left subsclavian artery to below the renal arteries; a separate graft was inserted to the left renal artery. The aneurysm had ruptured just above the diaphragm into a very large hiatal hernia sac.

The patient who died in hospital had undergone surgical treatment of an acute Type I aortic dissection by composite valve graft replacement of his ascending aorta elsewhere in 1989. The operation was complicated by previous pectus excavatum repair. The patient developed a sternal wound infection secondary to *Staphylococcus epidermidis.* One year later this patient developed severe left ventricular failure and was found to have a large perivalvular leak and a pseudoaneurysm. Bacterial endocarditis was diagnosed and initially treated with intravenous antibiotics followed by re-operation and primary repair of the perivalvular leak along with direct reimplantation of coronary arteries. Seven months later he again developed bacterial endocarditis and suffered an intracerebral hemorrhage resulting in a dense left hemiplegia. One year following the second operation he again developed congestive heart failure. Once again, a large false aneurysm surrounding his composite valve graft, secondary to a recurrent dehiscence of the aortic valve annulus, had developed. Two-thirds of the prosthetic valve annulus had separated from the native valve annular tissues. He was referred for surgical treatment. Operation involved resection and re-replacement of the entire composite valve graft. A viable omentum pedicle flap was placed in the mediastinum for coverage of the aortic graft. The patient suffered sudden death secondary to cardiac arrhythmias 2 weeks following operation.

Two late deaths occurred 6 months and 3 years after operation. Causes of late deaths were respiratory insufficiency in one and complications from AIDS in another. The patient who died from AIDS was HIV-positive at the time of aortic surgery.

Discussion

The Marfan syndrome is a disorder of connective tissue, which is generally inherited in an autosomal dominant manner with varying degrees of expressivity and penetrance. The current estimate of prevalence for Marfan syndrome is 1 in 20 000 (1). Patients with the disorder have a shortened life expectancy with a mean age approximating 32 years (2). The most common cause of death continues to be secondary to the cardiovascular manifestations of the disease, primarily aortic dissection and aneurysm rupture (12). Timely operative intervention often requiring multiple staged procedures favorably affects long-term survival (13). Diffuse dilatation of the proximal segment of the ascending aorta producing subsequent aortic annular dilatation and consequently aortic valvular insufficiency is the most common cardiovascular manifestation. Separate replacement of the aortic valve and ascending aorta results in aneurysmal dilatation of the sinus segment. The single most important contribution to the treatment of such patients was by Bentall and DeBono who first reported upon a successful composite valve graft replacement of the aortic root (11, 14). In their approach the aortic aneurysm wall is wrapped around the composite graft for purposes of hemostasis.

Kouchoukos and associates reported upon an experience with 127 patients requiring composite valve graft insertion. 103 underwent the classical Bentall-DeBono technique with the aortic wall wrapped around the composite valve graft. The most recent 24 patients in their series underwent an open button technique for reattachment of the coronary artery origins. Intraoperative hemorrhage and the development of early and late pseudoaneurysm formation was markedly reduced in those patients treated by button technique (15). Tension and lack of access to suture lines is the most frequent source of troublesome intraoperative bleeding and late pseudoaneurysm formation. Cabrol suggested interposing a transversely positioned smaller Dacron tube graft off of the aortic graft to the aorta around the coronary artery origins as a method of relieving such tension (16).

We have applied composite valve graft replacement to all patients with Marfan syndrome undergoing operation upon the aortic valve and/or ascending aorta (17/18). In our experience in patients both with and without Marfan syndrome requiring composite valve graft replacement, we have encountered difficulties with the classic Bentall operation similar to those described above. In all patients undergoing first-time operations and under any applicable circumstances, we preferentially employ the open "button" technique allowing for direct tension-free reattachment of the coronary artery origins to the aortic graft (Fig. 1). In patients undergoing redo operations and in selected patients with dissection and/or large aneurysms where mobilization of the coronary artery origins is neither practical nor feasible, the Cabrol operation or similar modification is employed (19). In this series, 21 patients required insertion of composite valve grafts. Thirteen patients underwent primary aortic root replacement not having had prior cardiac surgery. Eight patients who underwent composite insertion had had prior cardiac surgery. Of the 13 patients undergoing primary composite insertion, the open "button" technique was utilized in 12 and the Cabrol operation in 1. In the 8 patients undergoing redo operation, the Cabrol operation was used in 7 patients and the open "button" technique in 1.

In patients presenting with simple annulo-aortic ectasia without dissection, generally ascending aortic replacement with composite valve graft is adequate. In 1 of our 9 patients (44.4%) with dissecting ascending aortic aneurysms (all four with chronic dissection), we performed arch replacement in addition to ascending aortic composite valve graft replacement (Table 2). However, in patients with acute aortic dissection, the operation is carried out using hypothermia and circulatory arrest for an open distal anastomosis both to examine the arch for any additional tears which may need repair or excision and to obliterate the false lumen in the distal suture line. Aneurysmal dilatation of the arch, either fusiform or from dissection, likewise requires replacement using circulatory arrest.

Table 2: Current aortic operations for dissections and nondissections

Aortic operations	Dissection (n = 38)	Nondissection (n = 21)	Total
Ascending			
composite valve graft	5	12	17
false aneurysm repair	–	3	3
redo composite valve graft	–	3	3
Transverse arch grafting	1	–	1
Ascending + arch	4	–	4
Composite + arch	4	–	4
Descending	6	1	7
Thoracoabdominal	20	2	22
Descending + thoracoabdominal	1	–	1
Coarctation repair	–	1	1
Abdominal aortic aneurysm	2	1	3
Total	43	23	66

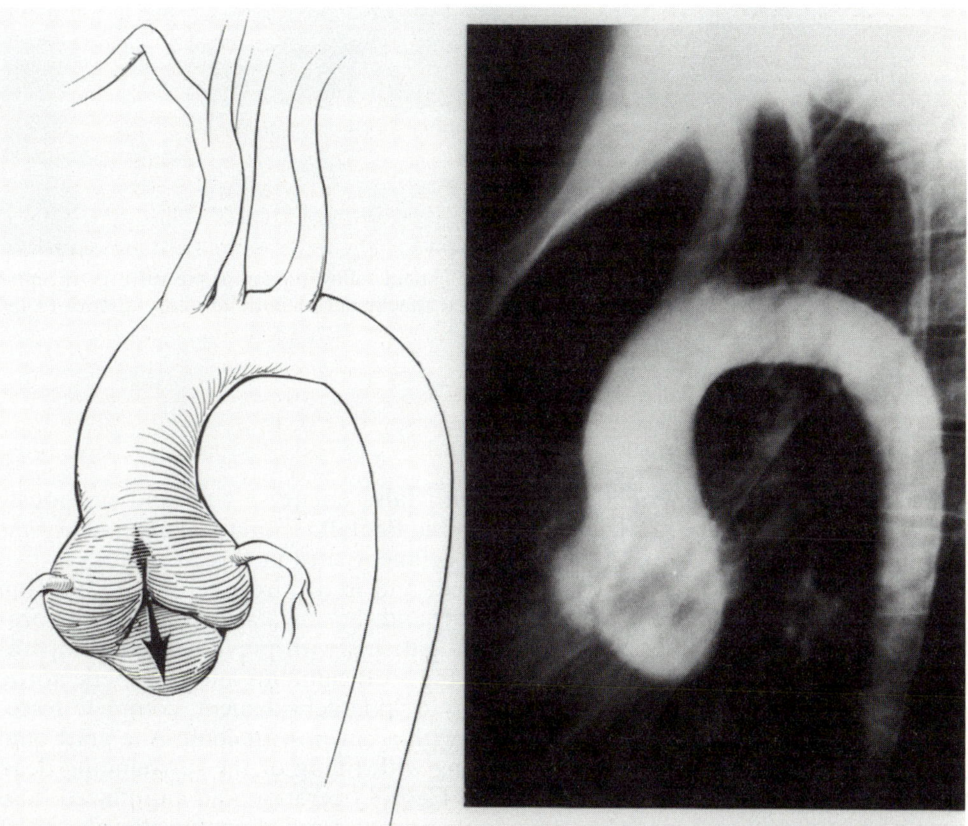

Fig. 1. A) Arteriogram and drawing of patient with annulo-aortic ectasia and moderate aortic valvular insufficiency.

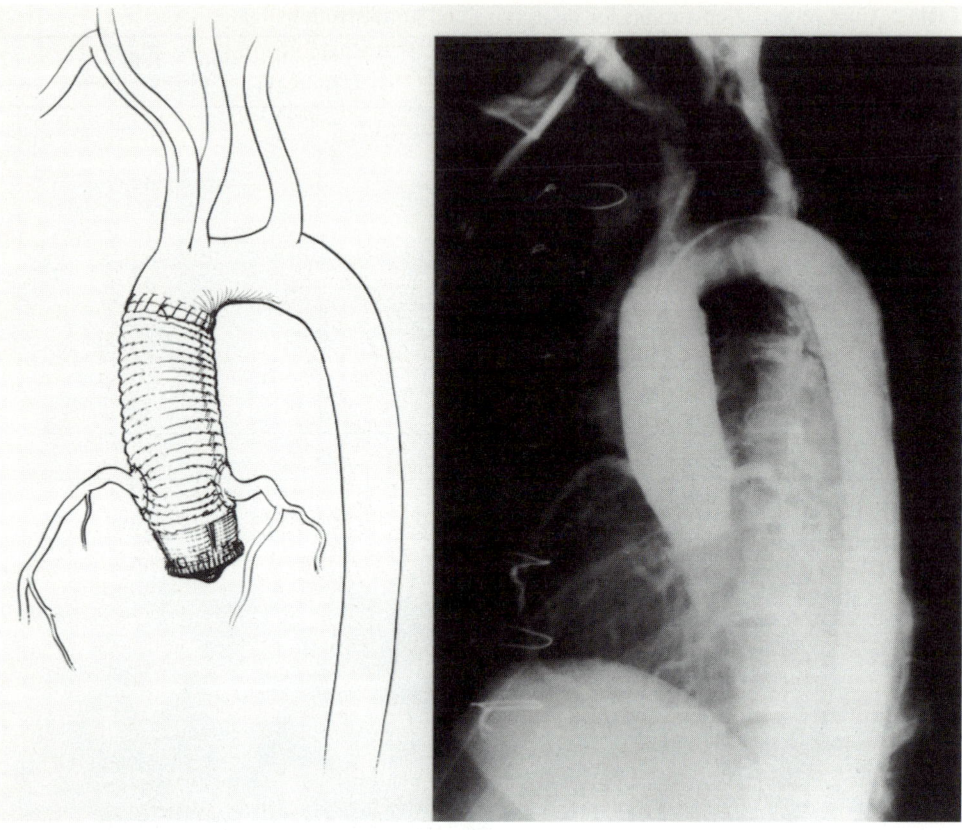

Fig. 1. B) Postoperative drawing and aortogram of patient following composite valve graft repair of the aortic root and ascending aorta with direct reattachment of both coronary arteries to the graft.

Five patients in this series presented with false aneurysms around previously inserted composite valve grafts using the classic Bentall technique. False aneurysms originated from right coronary artery reattachment sites in three patients. In two of them direct primary repair was employed, and in a third one an interposition graft of Dacron (between the composite graft and the aorta around the right coronary artery origin) was utilized. In the two patients with previous Bentall operations, the false aneurysms were localized to the aortic annulus and prosthetic aortic material involved with infection. We employed wide debridement, complete resection of all foreign material, re-replacement with a new in-situ composite graft, and viable tissue coverage of graft material along with filling of the surrounding dead space. Also, for one patient with a previous Cabrol operation and an infected false aneurysm originating from the aortic annulus, we performed composite valve graft re-replacement. Omentum was used in all these three patients with infected false aneurysms to cover the new composite grafts (21, 22).

Paraplegia remains one of the most devastating complications following resection and replacement of the descending thoracic or thoracoabdominal aorta (Fig. 2) (23–25). Only one patient in this series developed paraparesis and no patient developed paraplegia. The number of patients involved does not allow for statistical evaluation of techniques used and their relationship to outcome. In this series there

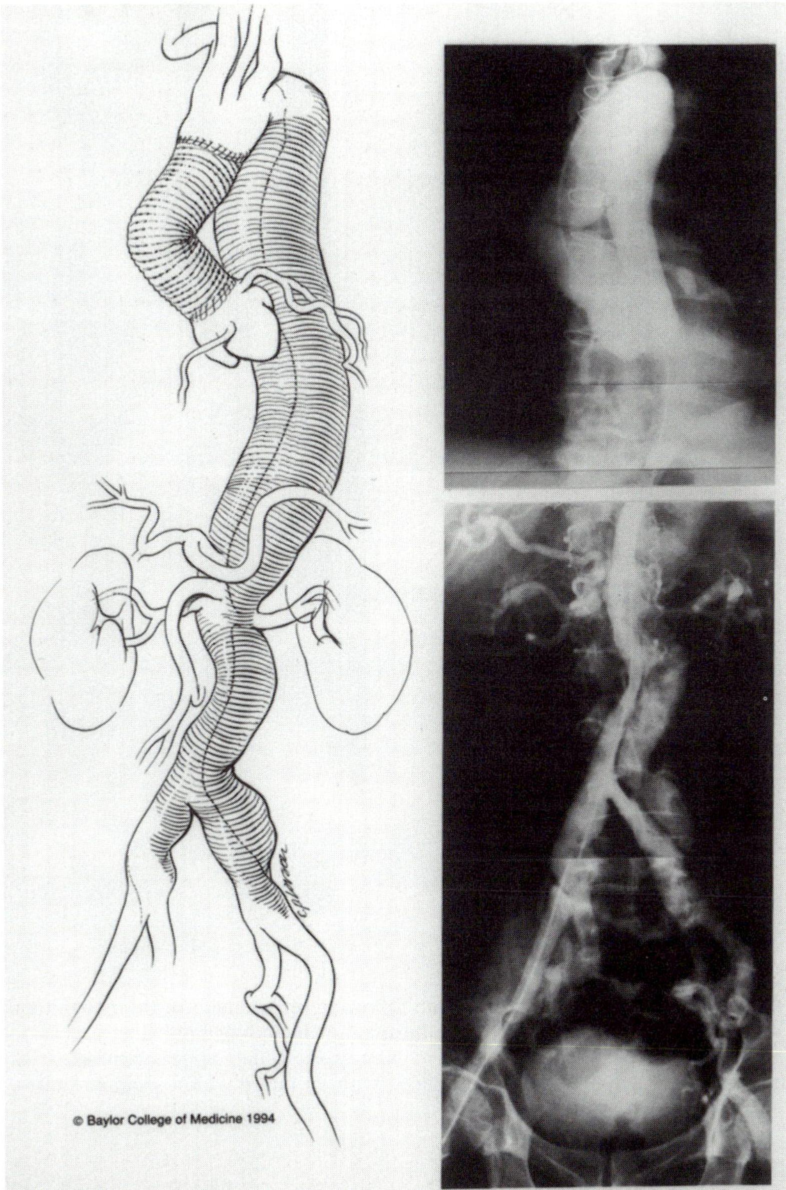

Fig. 2. A) Arteriogram and drawing of patient with extensive thoracoabdominal aortic aneurysm (extent II) with extension of dissection and aneurysmal involvement into both iliac arteries.

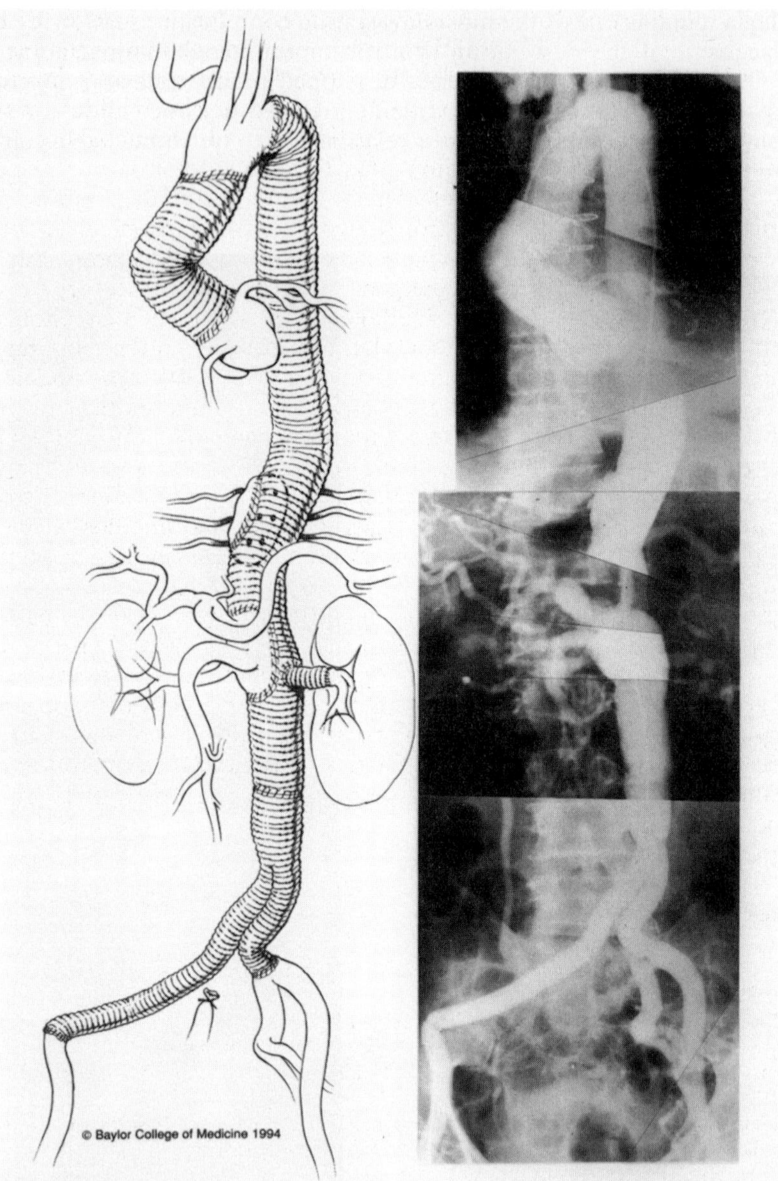

Fig. 2. B) Postoperative drawing and aortogram following replacement of thoracoabdominal aortic aneurysm from left subclavian artery to the bifurcation including both iliac arteries along with reattachment of multiple intercostal arteries as well as the celiac, superior mesenteric, and right renal arteries. The left renal artery was reattached with an interposition separate graft.

were 16 patients who underwent resection and graft replacement of distal aortic segments without the use of cardiofemoral bypass (descending thoracic aorta, 6 patients, and thoracoabdominal aorta, 10 patients). One of these requiring thoracoabdominal aortic replacement (Extent II – Crawford classification) was the patient who developed paraparesis. Thirteen patients (11 for thoracoabdominal aorta, 1 descending aorta, and 1 descending plus thoracoabdominal aorta) underwent resection and graft replacement of the descending thoracic aorta and/or the thoracoabdominal aorta using cardiofemoral bypass with a Biomedicus pump. All patients in which cardiofemoral bypass was used had dissection, and all were chronic except for 1 patient who emergently underwent replacement of the descending thoracic aorta for an acute DeBakey Type III aortic dissection. Another underwent replacement of the thoracoabdominal aorta from the diaphragm to the bifurcation (Extent IV) and descending thoracic aorta at the same operation using cardiofemoral bypass. In no instance was cerebrospinal fluid drainage or intrathecal papaverine used. In one patient femoro-femoral bypass and profound hypothermic circulatory arrest was used, because aortic size at the distal arch (12 cm) did not allow for placement of a clamp for proximal control. Cardiofemoral bypass was used to provide distal perfusion to the visceral vessels and intercostal arteries during the period of proximal anastomosis, which generally requires a longer period of time in the presence of dissection.

The variety and multiplicity of aortic operations in this group of patients with Marfan syndrome demonstrates the necessity for lifelong surveillance of remaining segments of unreplaced aorta as well as repaired segments for the future development of additional or recurrent aneurysm development. 117 aortic operations (66 current and 51 previous) in 59 patients is a strong indicator of the recurrent need for aortic surgery in patients with Marfan syndrome. Operative intervention in both instances can be undertaken with very satisfactory levels of morbidity and mortality.

References

1. Pyeritz RE, McKusick VA (1979) The Marfan syndrome: diagnosis and management. N Eng J Med 300: 772–779
2. Murdoch JL, Walker BA, Halpern BA, Kuzma JW, McKusick VA (1972) Life expectancy and causes of death in the Marfan Syndrome. N Eng J Med 286: 804–808
3. Magenis RE, Maslen CL, Smith L, Allen L, and Sakai LY (1991) Localization of the fibrillin (FBN) gene to Chromosome 15, Band q21.1 Genomics 11: 346–351
4. Kainulainen K, Steinmann B, Collins F, Dietz HC, Francomano CA, Child A, Kilpatrick MW, Brock DJH, Keston M, Pyeritz RE, Peltonen L (1991) Marfan syndrome: No evidence for heterogeneity in different populations, and more precise mapping of the gene. Am J Hum Genet 49: 662–667
5. Sakai LY, Keene DR, Glanville RW, Bächinger HP (1991) Purification and partial characterization of fibrillin, a Cysteine-rich structural component of connective tissue microfibrils. The Journal of Biological Chemistry 266: 14763–14770
6. Maslen CL, Corson GM, Maddox BK, Glanville RW, and Sakai LY (1991) Partial sequence of a candidate gene for the Marfan syndrome. Nature 352: 334–337
7. Lee B, Godfrey M, Vitale E, Hori H, Mattei M, Sarfarazi M, Tsipouras P, Ramirez F, and Hollister DW (1991) Linkage of Marfan syndrome and a phenotypically related disorder to two different fibrillin genes. Nature 352: 330–334
8. Franke U, Furthmayr H (1993) Genes and gene products involved in Marfan syndrome. Seminars in Thoracic and Cardiovasc Surg 5 (1): 3–10

9. Gerry JL Jr, Morris L, Pyeritz RE (1991) Clinical management of the cardiovascular complications of the Marfan syndrome. J State Med Soc 143 (3): 43–51
10. Crawford, ES, Crawford JL, Safi HJ, Coselli JS, Hess KR B. S., Brooks B A. R. T., Norton HJ, Glaeser DH D. Sc. (1986) Thoracoabdominal aortic aneurysms: preoperative and intraoperative factors determining immediate and long-term results of operations in 605 patients. J Vasc Surg 3: 389–404
11. Bentall H, DeBono A (1968) A technique for complete replacement of the ascending aorta. Thorax 23: 338
12. Habbal MHE (1992) Cardiovascular manifestations of Marfan's syndrome in the young. Am Heart J 123 (3): 253–257
13. Svensson LG, Crawford ES, Coselli JS, Safi HJ, Hess KR (1989) Impact of cardiovascular operation on survival in the Marfan patient. Supplement I Circulation 80: 233–242
14. Gott VL, Pyeritz RE, Cameron DE, Greene PS, McKusick VA (1911) Composite graft repair of Marfan aneurysm of the ascending aorta: results in 100 patients. Ann Thorac Surg 52: 38–45
15. Kouchoukos NT, Marshall WG Jr, Wedige-Stecher TA (1986) Eleven-year experience with composite graft replacement of the ascending aorta and aortic valve. J Thorac Cardiovasc Surg 92: 691–705
16. Cabrol C, Pavie A, Mesnildrey P, et al (1986) Long-term results with total replacement of the ascending aorta and reimplantation of the coronary arteries. J Thorac Cardiovasc Surg 91: 12
17. Svensson LG, Crawford ES, Hess KR, Coselli JS, Safi HJ (1992) Composite valve graft replacement of the proximal aorta: comparison of techniques in 348 patients. An Thorac Surg 54: 427–39
18. Coselli JS, Crawford ES (1993) Composite aortic valve replacement and graft replacement of the ascending aorta plus coronary ostial reimplantation: how I do it. Sem Thor Cardiovasc Surg 5 (1): 55–62
19. Coselli JS, Crawford ES (1989) Composite valve graft replacement of aortic root using separate Dacron tube for coronary artery reattachment. Ann Thorac Surg 47: 558–65
20. Crawford ES, Coselli JS (1988) Marfan syndrome: combined composite valve graft replacement of the aortic root and transaortic mitral valve replacement. Ann Thor Surg 45: 296–302
21. Coselli JS, Crawford ES, Williams TW Jr, Bradshaw MW, Wiemer DR, Harris RL, Safi HJ (1990) Treatment of postoperation infection of ascending aorta and transverse aortic arch, including use of viable omentum and muscle flaps. Ann Thor Surg 50: 868–881
22. Chan FY, Crawford ES, Coselli JS, Safi HJ, William TW Jr (1989) In-situ prosthetic graft replacement for mycotic aneurysms of the aorta. Ann Thorac Surg 47: 193–202
23. Crawford ES, Svensson LG, Hess KR, Shenaq SS, Coselli JS, Safi HJ, Mohindra PK, Rivera V (1991) A prospective randomized study of cerebrospinal fluid drainage to prevent paraplegia after high-risk surgery on the thoracoabdominal aorta. J Vasc Surg 13: 36–46
24. Coselli JS (1992) Suprarenal aortic reconstruction: endovascular repair. Sem Vasc Surg 5 (3): 180–191
25. Svensson LG, Crawford ES, Hess KR, Coselli JS, Safi HJ (1993) Experience with 1509 patients undergoing thoracoabdominal aortic operations. J Vasc Surg 17 (2): 357–70

Authors' address:
Joseph S. Coselli, M. D.
6535 Fannin, M. S. B405
Houston, TX 77030
USA

Aortic disease in Marfan syndrome: surgery, results, and special aspects

M. K. Heinemann, B. Buehner, M. J. Jurmann, J. Laas, H. G. Borst

Division of Thoracic and Cardiovascular Surgery, Surgical Center, Hannover Medical School, Hannover, FRG

Introduction

Marfan syndrome is a hereditary disorder of the connective tissue. Due to genetic determination by a mutation localized on chromosome 15, pathological fibrillin, an essential structural protein of elastic fibers, is synthesized. This leads to a disarray of fibers with resultant hyperelasticity and weakness. The expression of the disease is pleiomorphic, but in general it affects the ocular, skeletal and/or cardiovascular systems. The complications of cardiovascular manifestations, in particular aortic aneurysmatic dilatation and dissection without arterial hypertension and at an early age, have for a long time been limiting the life expectancy of these patients to about 40 years (8, 12, 19, 20). With the introduction of Bentall's technique for composite aortic root replacement, significant improvements for Marfan patients could be achieved. This was especially the case if they were operated upon electively, usually before the diameter of the ascending aorta reached 6 cm (9).

This paper reviews our experience with the treatment of aortic disease in Marfan syndrome over a 13-year time-span.

Study Population

Between January 1979 and August 1993, 95 patients were treated at Hannover Medical School for aortic disease in association with Marfan Syndrome. All patients met the diagnostic criteria as defined in the Berlin nosology (2). There was a preponderance of males (61 males, 34 females), with an average age of 35.5 years (range: 12 to 68 years). This mean age is 10 years below that of all patients treated for thoracic aortic disease at our institution.

The distribution of aortic disease is shown in Table 1. A quarter of all patients presented with aneurysm of the ascending aorta, and three quarters had some form of aortic dissection.

Operative Strategy

Indications for replacement of the *ascending aorta* were: acute type A aortic dissection, ascending aortic aneurysm or chronic type A aortic dissection with a diameter of 5 cm or more, and severe aortic valve regurgitation. Rapid progression of an ectatic aortic diameter less than 5 cm was also an indication for elective ascending

Table 1. Distribution of aortic disease in Marfan syndrome

Aortic disease	Abbreviation	Number of Patients	Percentage
acute type A aortic dissection	AADA	26	24.7%
chronic type A aortic dissection	CADA	29	27.6%
acute type B aortic dissection	AADB	5	4.8%
chronic type B aortic dissection	CADB	9	8.6%
ascending aortic aneurysm	ANEU	26	24.7%

aortic replacement, especially in the younger patients with known Marfan syndrome who were followed regularly by their cardiologist.

In the 81 patients with a primarily affected *ascending aorta,* composite graft replacement of the aortic valve and ascending aorta with reimplantation of the coronaries was the procedure most frequently performed (n = 66). In 12 patients, the aortic valve could be retained and the ascending aorta was replaced above the coronaries. Two patients underwent reconstruction of the ascending aorta early during the experience. One patient presented with chronic type A aortic dissection and aneurysmatic dilatation of his dissected descending thoracic aorta exceeding 8 cm, so that descending aortic replacement was performed as a first measure.

In 17 of the 55 patients (= 31%) with either acute of chronic type A aortic dissection, surgery was extended into the *aortic arch,* utilizing deep hypothermic circulatory arrest. A proximal arch replacement was performed in six (three acute, three chronic). Total aortic arch replacement with reimplantation of the head vessels was done in 11 cases (three acute, eight chronic). In four instances of chronic dissection with considerable distal aortic pathology, an elephant trunk was inserted into the downstream descending thoracic aorta (3).

Fourteen patients presented with a primarily affected *descending thoracic aorta:* five with acute and nine with chronic type B aortic dissection. A diameter of more than 6 cms or rapid enlargement were regarded as indications for elective aortic replacement. Primary therapy for acute type B aortic dissection in our institution is antihypertensive. The patient is transferred to surgery if there is (impending) aortic rupture, malperfusion of vital organs or persisting pain despite normotension. In 12 patients replacement of the descending thoracic aorta through a left thoracotomy and utilizing partial left atrial – femoral arterial bypass was performed (4). One patient with acute type B aortic dissection developed retrograde extension of her intimal tear under medical treatment, eventually leading to aortic valve insufficiency. She thus converted to a type A dissection and underwent emergency composite graft replacement. One other patient with chronic type B aortic dissection with a diameter of 6.5 cm suffered from concomitant non-dissected ascending aortic aneurysm with III° aortic valve regurgitation. Therefore, he was first subjected to composite graft replacement, followed by descending aortic replacement 8 weeks later.

Results

Early mortality, i.e., within 30 days of operation or never having left the hospital, was 7.4% (7/95) overall. It was highest in the acute type A dissection group (4/26 = 15.6%) and lowest in acute as well as chronic type B dissection (0/14 = 0%). This latter result may be biased by the comparatively small number. Late mortality was highest in chronic type A dissection (4/27 survivors = 14.8%) and lowest in the patients with annuloaortic ectasia (1/25 survivors = 4%). The mortalities according to the diagnosis at first presentation are listed in Table 2.

Causes of death are given in Table 3. There were three deaths (one early, two late) from aortic complications, i.e., rupture or malperfusion of vital organs. The majority of lethal complications was of a cardiopulmonary nature. One patient with severe mitral regurgitation died from a ventricular arrhythmia awaiting mitral valve repair.

Reoperations

There was a total of 39 reoperations in 29 out of 79 patients surviving the primary procedure. Indications for reoperations were increasingly dilated aortic diameter,

Table 2. Early and late mortality

	Early mortality	Late mortality
Overall	7/95 (= 7.4%)	9/88 (= 10.2%)
AADA	4/26 (= 15.4%)	2/22 (= 13.6%)
CADA	2/29 (= 6.9%)	4/27 (= 14.8%)
AADB/CADB	0/14 (= 0%)	1/14 (= 7.1%)
ANEURYSM	1/26 (= 3.8%)	1/25 (= 4%)

Table 3: Causes of death (early/late)

	AADA	CADA	ANEURYSM
Cardiopulmonary	2/2	0/0	1/1
Sepsis	1/0	0/2	0/0
CNS	0/0	1/1	0/0
Technical	1/0	0/0	0/0
Aortic	0/1	1/1	0/0
Suicide	0/0	0/1	0/0

Table 4. Location of reoperations

	AADA	CADA	AADB	CADB	ANEU
ASC	1	1	3	1	2
ARCH	3	0	0	0	0
DESC	6	5	0	0	1
TH-ABD	3	3	2	5	0
ABD	2	1	0	0	0

asc = ascending aorta; arch = aortic arch; desc = descending thoracic aorta; th-abd = thoraco-abdominal aorta; abd = abdominal aorta

Table 5. Distribution and outcome of reoperations

Diagnosis	Operations	Patients	Early mort.	Late mort.	Survival
AADA	15	10	2	1	70%
CADA	10	7	1	0	86%
AADB	5	4	0	0	100%
CADB	6	5	1	0	80%
ANEU	3	3	0	0	100%
total	= 39	= 29	= 4	= 1	= 83%

usually more than 6 cm, malperfusion of vital organs, or a failed primary operation. Location and outcome of the reoperative procedures are given in Tables 4 and 5.

The reoperation rate was significantly higher in patients who had an already dissected aorta at the time of their first operation (36 reoperations in 26/55 surviving patients = 47.2% of survivors) when compared to the group with isolated aneurysm of the ascending aorta (three reoperations in 3/24 surviving patients = 12.5% of survivors).

The elephant trunk technique to facilitate staged reintervention was utilized in 10 reoperations: one aortic arch and nine descending thoracic aortic replacements.

Discussion

The problem of when to replace a dilated aorta in a patient with Marfan Syndrome has been a vexing one for many years. The Johns Hopkins group was able to achieve good results by drawing the line for elective replacement of the ascending aorta at 6 cm (9). Thus, they were able to prevent aortic dissection which in turn has led to very good late outcome. Pyeritz showed that in patients with a family history of aortic dissection this event may occur even in aortas with a diameter of less than 5 cm, suggesting earlier elective operation (19). There are no hard data in the scarce literature on the issue of the critical aortic diameter, but several groups accepting 5 to 6 cm as an indication for aortic replacement were able to achieve good long-term survival (5, 10, 16, 22).

If our material is analyzed over time, there is an increasing number of arch procedures during primary operation for type A dissection. Growing experience with deep hypothermic circulatory arrest has rendered this to be a safe method for cerebral protection, not increasing the risk of ascending aortic surgery (11, 17). A more radical primary operation may obviate the need for reintervention in the long term (1, 6, 15, 18).

The location of reoperations follows certain patterns according to the primary diagnosis. Patients with type A dissection undergo ascending aortic repair as a first procedure. Their most frequent site of reoperation is the descending aorta. Reoperations upon the aortic arch have been avoided so far in chronic type A dissection, probably due to a very radical approach during the primary operation with concomitant total arch replacement in 8 out of 28 ascending aortic procedures.

In acute type B dissection there is the danger of ante- as well as retrograde extension of the disease, with three reoperations having become necessary upon the ascending aorta, and two on the thoracoabdominal portion. In the chronic type B variant downstream dilatation or malperfusion led to a majority of reoperations on the thoracoabdominal aorta.

Reoperations after elective replacement of the ascending aorta for aneurysm are rare and have mostly been confined to the repair of unsatisfactory primary procedures. One patient underwent unsuccessful aortic valve resuspension early during the experience and had to be reoperated with composite graft replacement. One patient underwent reoperation for perfused graft inclusion after composite replacement. In one other patient development of a second aneurysm necessitated descending aortic replacement.

Meticulous long-term follow-up is necessary to determine progression of aortic dilatation in time. We have instituted our own database and the schedule of necessary investigations is organized by the surgeon (10). Computed tomography scanning is the method of choice for assessing aortic pathology, supplemented by transesophageal echocardiography. Digital subtraction angiography is only necessary for evaluation of questionable organ perfusion. Magnetic resonance imaging helps to reduce radiation exposure, but is still expensive and of limited availability.

In so-called annuloaortic ectasia and mild to moderate aortic valve regurgitation the question of valve replacement versus reconstruction has been discussed repeatedly. As the patients with the Marfan Syndrome are generally young, the contraindications for mechanical valve prostheses with anticoagulation are legion. We have recently begun to preserve the aortic valve in elective ascending aortic replacement, utilizing both the techniques described by Yacoub (21) and David (7). As the follow-up of these patients is still too short, their data are not included in this series. Early results, however, are very encouraging.

Discussion of non-cardiac aspects

Several non-cardiac manifestations of Marfan Syndrome are of considerable importance for the planning of and care after an aortic procedure.

Most patients have skeletal deformities due to their connective tissue disease.

Scoliosis of the thoracic spine may lead to heart displacement, rendering access to the aorta difficult. It can also cause prolonged respiratory problems during post-operative care.

A frequent chest wall deformity in patients with Marfan syndrome is *funnel chest*. This, again may lead to shifting of the heart into the left hemithorax and awkward access to the aorta. In known aortic dilatation two-stage repair should be considered with the funnel chest correction as the primary procedure before elective intervention on the aorta. Methods for rapid staged repair in urgent cases have been described (14, 23).

Weakness of the connective tissue of the lung may lead to bullous emphysema early in life. Recurrent *pneumothoraces* with long-lasting drainage treatment are known complications after thoracic procedures in patients with Marfan syndrome (13).

Conclusions

From the above analysis we draw the following conclusions for treatment of aortic disease in patients with the Marfan syndrome:

1) The risks and rate of reoperations are significantly higher if the patients have already dissected at the time of their primary procedure.

2) Prophylactic replacement of a dilated ascending aorta is therefore recommended. A diameter of 5 cm in the ascending and 6 cm in the descending aorta is regarded as the cut-off point.

3) Non-cardiac manifestations may adversely affect the cardiovascular procedures.

4) Only appropriate primary surgery and meticulous long-term follow-up can achieve satisfactory results.

References

1. Bachet J, Teodori G, Goudot B, et al. (1988) Replacement of the transverse aortic arch during emergency operations for type A acute aortic dissection: report of 26 cases. J Thorac Cardiovasc Surg 96: 878–886
2. Beighton P, dePaepe A, Danks D, et al. (1988) International nosology of heritable disorders of connective tissue Berlin 1986. Am J Med Genet 29: 581–594
3. Borst HG, Frank G, Schaps D (1988) Treatment of extensive aortic aneurysms by a new multiple-stage approach. J Thorac Cardiovasc Surg 95: 11–13
4. Borst HG, Jurmann MJ, Bühner B, Laas J (1994) Risk of replacement of descending aorta with a standardized left heart bypass technique. J Thorac Cardiovasc Surg 107: 126–133
5. Crawford ES, Coselli JS, Svensson LG, Safi HJ, Hess KR (1990) Diffuse aneurysmal disease (chronic aortic dissection, Marfan, and megaaorta syndromes) and multiple aneurysm. Ann Surg 211: 521–537
6. Crawford ES, Kirklin JW, Naftel DC, et al (1992) Surgery for acute dissection of the ascending aorta: should the arch be included? J Thorac Cardiovasc Surg 104: 46–59
7. David TE, Feindel CM (1992) An aortic valve-sparing operation for patients with aortic incompetence and aneurysm of the ascending aorta. J Thorac Cardiovasc Surg 103: 617–622
8. Francke U, Furthmayr H (1993) Genes and gene products involved in Marfan Syndrome. Sem Thorac Cardiovasc Surg 5: 3–10
9. Gott VL, Pyeritz RE, Cameron DE, Greene PS, McKusick VA (1991) Composite graft repair of Marfan aneurysm of the ascending aorta: results in 100 patients. Ann Thorac Surg 52: 38–45

10. Heinemann MK, Laas J, Karck M, Borst HG (1990) Thoracic aortic aneurysms after acute type A aortic dissection: necessity for follow-up. Ann Thorac Surg 49: 580–584
11. Heinemann MK, Laas J, Jurmann MJ, Karck M, Borst HG (1991) Surgery extended into the aortic arch in acute type A aortic dissection: indications, techniques, results. Circulation 84 (suppl III): 25–30
12. Hirata K, Triposkiadis F, Sparks E, et al (1991) The Marfan Syndrome: abnormal elastic properties. JACC 18: 57–63
13. Hirata K, Triposkiadis F, Sparks E, et al (1992) The Marfan Syndrome: cardiovascular physical findings and diagnostic correlates. Am Heart J 123: 743–752
14. Jones WG, Hoffman L, Devereux RB, Isom OW, Gold JP (1994) Staged approach to combined repair of pectus excavatum and lesions of the heart. Ann Thorac Surg 57: 212–214
15. Kirklin JW, Kouchoukos NT (1993) When and how to include arch repair in patients with acute dissections involving the ascending aorta. Sem Thorac Cardiovasc Surg 5: 27–32
16. Kouchoukos NT, Marshall WG (1986) Treatment of ascending aortic dissection in the Marfan Syndrome. J Cardiac Surg 1: 333–346
17. Laas J, Jurmann MJ, Heinemann MK, Borst HG (1992) Advances in aortic arch surgery. Ann Thorac Surg 53: 227–232
18. Lansman SL, Raissi S, Ergin A, Griepp RB (1989) Urgent operation for acute transverse aortic arch dissection. J Thorac Cardiovasc Surg 97: 334–341
19. Pyeritz RE (1993) Marfan Syndrome: current and future clinical and genetic management of cardiovascular manifestations. Sem Thorac Cardiovasc Surg 5: 11–16
20. Roberts WC, Honig HS (1982) The spectrum of cardiovascular disease in the Marfan Syndrome: a clinico-morphologic study of 18 necropsy patients. Am Heart J 104: 115–135
21. Sarsam MAI, Yacoub M (1993) Remodeling of the aortic valve anulus. J Thorac Cardiovasc Surg 105: 435–438
22. Svensson LG, Crawford ES, Coselli JS, Safi HJ, Hess KR (1989) Impact of cardiovascular operation on survival in the Marfan patient. Circulation 80 (suppl I): 233–242
23. Tschirkov A, Natschev G, Miskev B, Savova A, Ovanessjan H (1989) An easy and safe approach for simultaneous repair of severe pectus excavatum and the underlying lesions of the heart and thoracic aorta. J Thorac Cardiovasc Surg 98: 305–307

Authors' address:
Dr. med. M. Heinemann
Klinik für Thorax-, Herz- und Gefäßchirurgie
Medizinische Hochschule Hannover
Konstanty-Gutschow-Str. 8
30625 Hannover
FRG

Results of cardiovascular surgery for Marfan syndrome in Berlin

R. Hetzer, P. Gehle, J. Ennker

German Heart Institute Berlin, Department of Cardiothoracic and Vascular Surgery, Berlin, FRG

Marfan patients who have undergone surgery at the German Heart Institute Berlin included patients who met the diagnostic criteria for Marfan syndrome as established at the Conference on International Nosology of Heritable Disorders of Connective Tissue held in Berlin in 1986 (1, 25) and so-called "marfanoid" patients, i.e., patients who exhibited typical manifestations in three different organ systems (cardiovascular, ocular, skeletal, or other organ systems) while not completely fulfilling the diagnostic criteria for Marfan syndrome (22).

Indication and type of surgery

As of May 1994, we have performed 148 operations in 135 patients since the inception of our institution in April 1986. Seventy-seven patients were diagnosed as having Marfan syndrome and 58 as exhibiting marfanoid manifestations. The patients, including 103 males and 32 females, ranged in age from 9 to 65 years with a mean age of 38.7 years. Indications for surgery are listed in Table 1 whereby a distinction is made between elective and emergency operations. There were 73 elective operations for aneurysms and/or aortic valve incompetence and 33 operations for mitral valve incompetence. We also had 35 emergency operations for dissection and/or rupture, one for mitral valve incompetence, and six for cardiac failure.

In 24 patients it became necessary to operate in the same region of the previous surgery: ten for aneurysms of the ascending aorta and the aortic arch, nine for aneurysms and/or dissections of the descending and abdominal aorta and peripheral vessels, five for mitral incompetence, and three for the management of myocardial failure (Table 1). A typical reason for subsequent re-intervention was the implantation of a prosthesis in the ascending aorta which was too short and thus allowed recurrent aneurysm formations proximal or distal to the graft. Various surgical techniques have been described for ascending aortic replacements in Marfan patients (2, 3, 6, 7, 8, 15, 16, 18). We performed composite ascending and aortic valve replacement according to the Bentall (2) procedure 59 times, and according to the Cabrol (7) procedure 22 times. A combination of both techniques was used in two patients (Table 2). In the early phase of our program a few patients underwent separate replacement of the aortic valve and the supracoronary ascending aorta or wrapping of the ascending aorta. Two patients underwent only aortic valve replacement. More recently, four patients underwent replacement of the ascending aorta with preservation of the aortic valve. Additionally, one patient underwent

Table 1. Indications for surgery

Elective operations for aneurysms and/or aortic valvular incompetence	73
Mitral valvular incompetence	33
	106
Emergency operations for dissection and/or rupture	35
Mitral valve incompetence	1
Cardiac failure	6
	42
Reoperations for aneurysms of the ascending aorta and aortic arch	10
Aneurysm and/or dissection of distal aortic segments and peripheral vessels	9
Mitral valve incompetence	5
	24

Table 2. Type of Operation

A	Composite replacement of the ascending aorta and aortic valve		
	Bentall		59
	Cabrol		22
	one side Bentall on side Cabrol		2
			83
	Separate replacement of aortic valve and of the ascending aorta		6
	Aortic valve replacement and wrapping of the ascending aorta		5
	Replacement of the ascending aorta with preservation of the native aortic valve		4
	Aortic valve replacement		2
			17
B	Aortic arch replacement		1
	Replacement of the descending aorta		7
	Thoraco-abdominal replacement		2
	Infrarenal aortic replacement		1
			11
C	Mitral valve repair		
	Gerbode		15
	Paneth		4
	Combination of individual reconstruction procedures		12
	(Including posterior annulus reinforcement)	(8)	
	Mitral valve replacement		11
	(Including mitral valve replacement after reconstruction)	(5)	
			42
D	Tricuspid valve repair		
	DeVega		5
	Kay		6
			11

aortic arch replacement. The descending thoracic aorta was replaced in seven patients, the thoracoabdominal aorta in two, and the infrarenal segment in one.

Mitral and tricuspid valve surgery

Mitral valve surgery was performed in 42 cases. Mitral valvuloplasty was performed in 31 cases according to either the Gerbode (12) or Paneth (5) techniques, a combination of both, or individualized reconstructive procedures. Posterior annulus reinforcement using an autologous pericardial tissue flap was employed eight times. Mitral valve replacement was necessary 11 times including five patients who had undergone mitral reconstruction previously. Tricuspid valve repair was performed 11 times.

Preservation of the native aortic valve

Currently, replacement of the aortic root with preservation of the native aortic valve has been advocated in carefully selected patients with annulo-aortic ectasia or Marfan syndrome who have structurally sound aortic valve leaflets (9, 11, 26). This follows the concept of sparing the patient the well-known hazards of mechanical valve implantation, e.g. thromboembolism, prosthetic valve endocarditis, and the necessity of receiving anticoagulants. Although long-term results have not yet been determined, the initial results of other investigations have prompted us to perform ascending aortic replacement with a sinus-shaped graft with retention of the native aortic valve in three patients aged 9, 24, and 28. The prosthesis was cut in such a manner that the coronary orifice was left free and residual tissue was excluded (Fig. 1).

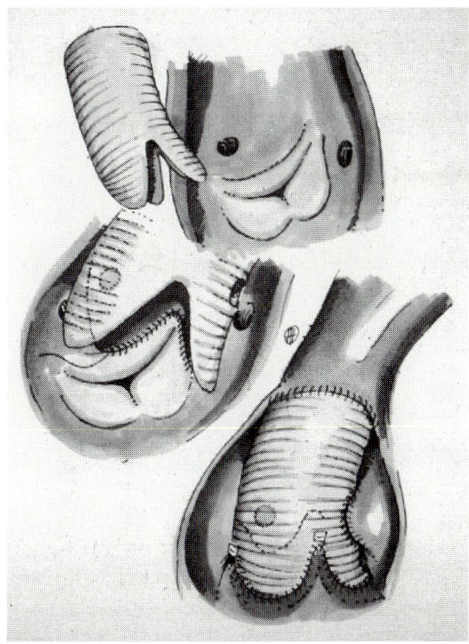

Fig. 1. Replacement of the aortic root and ascending aorta with preservation of the native aortic valve. The figure illustrates the steps used in implanting a sinusshaped prosthetic graft (Dacron of PTFE) with sutures to the aortic annulus and anastomoses of the coronary ostia to the graft in a Bentall-like fashion.

Table 3. Surgery for congestive heart failure

6 patients with endstage congestive heat faiture	
age: 15–42 years, mean 32	
sex: 6 males	
4 patients with Marfan Syndrome	
2 patients with marfanoid characteristics	
Implantation of a biventricular assist device (Berlin Heart)	5 pts.
Heart transplantation	4 pts. (3 after BVAD, 1 directly)

One patient died due to causes not related to the operation. A postoperative examination indicated no signs of myocardial infarction nor of valvular incompetence. The patient developed sepsis and multi-organ failure. The other two patients exhibited good postoperative function and continue to have a favorable follow-up.

Congestive heart failure

An unexpectedly high proportion of patients in the Marfan group presented with congestive heart failure due to myocardial dysfunction both primarily and during the follow-up period after previous cardiac or aortic operations. There were six

Table 4. Experience in the pediatric age group

30 Patients have been observed	
age: 4–15 years, mean 9.5 years	
sex: 16 females, 14 males	
Disease characteristics and manifestations	
Family history	27
Skeletal	30
Ocular	11
Aortic root dilatations	18
Mitral valve prolapse	17
3 patients have undergone surgery to date	
ages: 4, 12, 13 yrs	
sex: 2 females, 1 male	
aortic root dilatation in two:	
root diameter 3.8 cm and 6.5 cm	
acute aortic dissection with pericardial tamponade in one patient:	
root diameter 7.5 cm	
Operations performed	
Composite replacement of the ascending aorta and aortic valve	2
Replacement of the ascending aorta with preservation of the native aortic valve	1

such patients; in five heart failure was so advanced that it became necessary to implant a mechanical biventricular assist device system (Berlin Heart).

Two patients died due to complications during the assist period (thromboembolism and hemorrhaging) while three were supported until transplantation could be performed. One patient underwent transplantation directly. These four patients are presently in excellent condition.

Pediatric age group

Our experience in the pediatric age group is based upon treating 30 patients (see Table 4). Sixteen are females and 14 are males. They range in age from 4 to 15 years with a mean age of 9.5 years. Diagnosis was based on skeletal, ocular, and cardiovascular features and family history (17, 20, 24, 28). All subjects underwent echocardiography. Twenty-seven patients had a Marfan family history, 30 had skeletal abnormalities, 11 had ocular abnormalities, and 18 had aortic root dilatation. Seventeen patients had mitral valve prolapse. Follow-up studies consisted of transesophageal echocardiographic measurements of left ventricular diastolic and systolic function, valvular function of all four valves and five aortic diameters (annulus, aortic sinuses, sinu-tubular connection, arch distal of trunk origin, and the ascending aorta). Up to now surgery was performed on three of these patients, two females and one male, ages 4, 12, and 13 years, respectively. The indication was aortic root dilatation in two patients and an acute aortic dissection in one. This last patient, a 9-year-old boy, had an aortic diameter of 7.5 cm. Surgery consisted

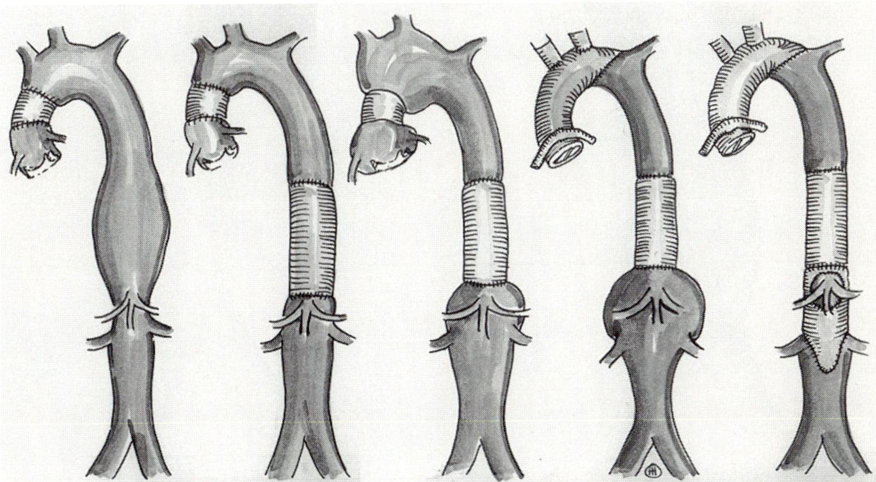

Fig. 2. Schematic drawings of several subsequent operations for aortic aneurysm formations in a typical Marfan patient:
Status upon admission, distal descending replacement (b), aortic valve, aortic root replacement (Cabrol), aortic arch replacement with side branches to supraaortic vessels (d), and thoraco-abdominal replacement with reattachment of the intestinal vessel (e).

of composite ascending and aortic valve replacement in two patients and replacement of the ascending aorta with preservation of the native aortic valve in another, a 9-year-old girl with an aortic dilatation of 3.8 cm (see Table 4).

Multiple operations

Among the 29 patients who had to be reoperated, there were two requiring multiple consecutive operations.

Patient 1: Prior to being treated at our facility, the patient had a short segment of prosthesis implanted in the ascending aorta and an aortic valve replacement with a biological prothesis. He later developed an aneurysm of the descending

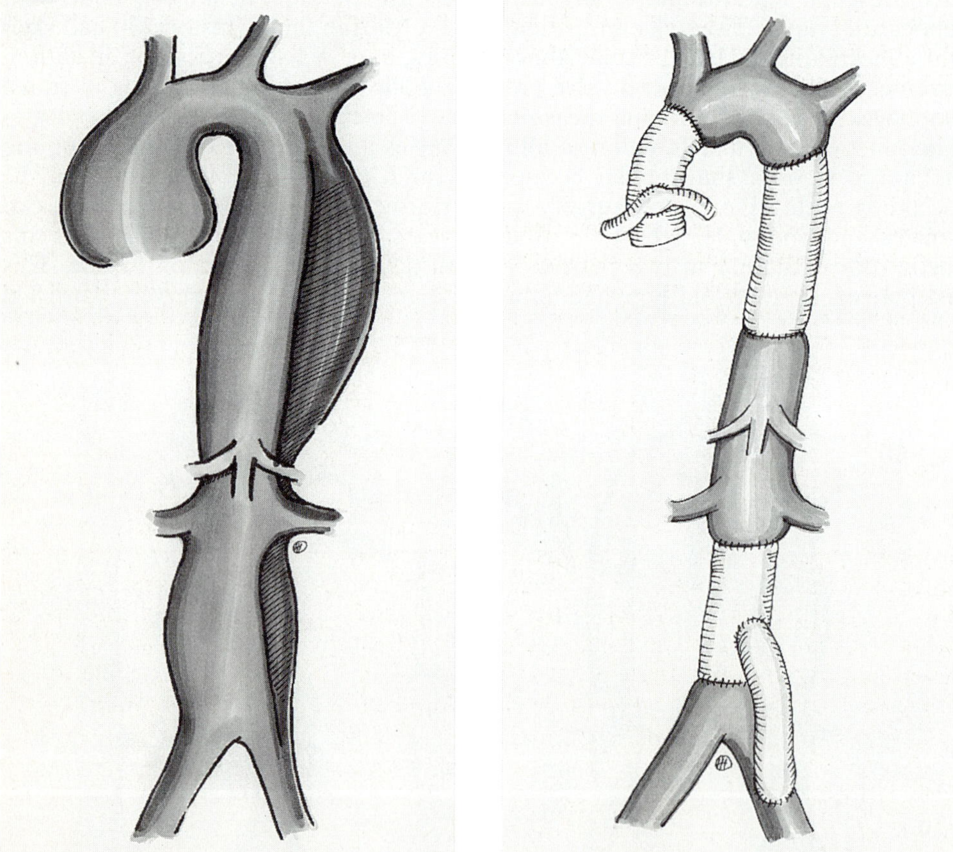

Fig. 3. Schematic drawings of consecutive surgery in a Marfan patient:
Status upon admission (left) with huge aneurysms of the ascending, descending, thoraco-abdominal, and infrarenal aorta with chronic dissection. Replacement of the ascending aorta and aortic root (Cabrol) (1), descending aorta (2), infrarenal aorta with a prosthetic bypass to the left iliac artery. After suffering congestive heart failure, the patient was supported with a biventricular assist device and subsequently underwent transplantation.

aorta. In 1991, we examined him for the first time and subsequently replaced his descending aorta. During the last 2 years the patient developed a large aneurysm of the aortic arch and of the supra-aortic vessels together with a suprarenal aortic aneurysm. He underwent reoperation a few months ago in which the ascending aorta, the aortic arch and the aortic valve were replaced by a composite graft and the brachiocephalic trunk and the left carotid artery were reattached via prosthetic side branches. Just recently, he underwent successful replacement of the suprarenal aortic segment (Fig. 2).

Patient 2: A 22-year-old typical Marfan patient had a huge aneurysm of both the ascending and descending aorta. The diameter of the ascending aorta reached 11 cm while that of the descending aorta, with a chronic type B dissection, reached 10 cm. All these segments were replaced consecutively within six months (Figure 3). Replacement of the infrarenal aorta and left common iliac artery was also necessary. After recovering from these operations, this patient developed congestive heart failure another two months later and had to be supported by a biventricular assist device (Berlin Heart). The patient was then successfully transplanted. Today, 6 months after undergoing cardiac transplantation, the patient is in good condition and has returned to work.

Results and follow-up

There were 13 early postoperative deaths (8.8%), three after elective surgery (2.8%) (sepsis, myocardial infarction, mediastinitis-sepsis) and ten following emergency surgery (24.3%) (Table 5). In our department the outcome of the majority of the patients (currently 96% of the entire group) is closely monitored during the follow-up period. Within 89 months there were 11 late deaths (81.%). Presently the actuarial survival rate is 86%).

Discussion

Cardiovascular manifestations of Marfan syndrome remain the leading cause of death in these patients. The results of a survey performed 22 years ago on the outcome of such patients showed that 72 of 257 patients had died and that 52 of the 56 patients with a known cause of death died due to causes related to the cardiovascular system. The mean age in this patient group was 32 years (18). This ominous prognosis has been restated by several reports (21, 23, 27). Due to improvements in early diagnosis, medical therapy, and surgical intervention, the life

Table 5. Results and follow-up

Early postoperative deaths	13	(8.8%)
in elective operations	3	(2.8%)
in emergency operations	10	(24.3%)
Late deaths	11	(8.1%)
Follow-up 1–89 months (mean: 34 months)		
Actuarial survival after 89 months	86%	

expectancy and quality of life of these patients has been gradually increased. In particular, the incidence of lethal complications, such as acute aortic dissection or rupture, could be reduced.

Although the indication for prophylactic aortic replacement continues to be debated, currently there is general consensus that surgical correction of aortic aneurysmal disease in adults should be surgically corrected if the diameter of the ascending aorta exceeds 5 cm or that of the descending aorta 6 cm. However, in patients with a family history of Marfan syndrome, a rapid expansion of the aorta over a short period of time is considered an indication for surgery. It is therefore extremely important to closely monitor the aortic diameters in these patients. Early surgery also has to be considered if there is a strong family history of aortic dissection at smaller diameters. While it is generally accepted that an acute dissection of the ascending aorta is an indication for emergency intervention, patients at our facility undergo surgery for dissection of the descending aorta only if complications develop or if aneurysm becomes evident. However, this policy has been questioned in particular by Miller (19) and may be reevaluated on the basis of longer follow-up (22).

Today, complete aortic root replacement using a composite graft, which was first described by Bentall in 1968 (2) and later modified, is the standard surgical procedure in Marfan patients. Incomplete replacement of the ascending aorta led to recurrent aortic root dilatation. Early reoperation was indicated in such cases to prevent the risk of subsequent rupture or dissection. Other reasons for reoperations several years after the primary procedure were a pseudoaneurysm orginating at the distal anastomosis in one patient and coronary ostial dilatation and dissection after composite replacement in two patients.

Early diagnosis includes regular transesophageal echocardiography or computed or magnetic nuclear resonance tomography follow-up examinations (4, 10). Total or partial aortic replacement may be performed using a multi-staged procedure which begins with the aortic segment of highest risk, usually the ascending aorta. Two patients underwent such a sequence of procedures at our facility without any postoperative neurologic deficits.

To avoid the long-term risks involved with combined mechanical valve replacement/composite graft insertion, Yacoub (26), David (9), and Ergin (11) initiated techniques for preserving the native aortic valve and resecting most of the aortic sinus tissue. We used a sinus-shaped graft which was inserted into the aorta and its edge sutured to the natural aortic annulus, thus preserving the native valve and stabilizing the aortic sinus area by excluding sinus tissue. The coronary ostia were reimplantated into the graft in a Bentell-type fashion. Valve competency was assessed by intraoperative transesophageal echocardiography. The significance of such valve-preserving procedures must be re-evaluated on the basis of long-term results in comparison with the well-established experience with composite valve-bearing prosthesis (15).

In our group of 135 patients, 42 (28% of all operations) underwent a mitral valve procedure either simultaneously (9 patients) with aortic replacement or separately in cases involving severe mitral insufficiency (33 patients). This incidence is consistent with the rate of 23% described by the Johns Hopkins group (13), which also reported an 80% feasibility of mitral valve reconstruction in patients with Marfan syndrome. In their 29 patients, four (14%) developed recurrent mitral regurgitation (grade III or IV) after previous repair: one subsequently underwent reoperation for endocarditis. We had to perform early reoperation in five of the 31 patients who had undergone primary repair (16%). These intermediate results demonstrate that the durability of mitral valve reconstruction is presently acceptable, however, not ideal. It must be anticipated that most, if not all preserved or reconstructed valves in these patients, be it in the aortic or the mitral position need to be replaced in the long-term eventually (14). Nevertheless, long-term follow-up of these patients is required in order to verify the current concept of mitral repair in cases of mitral regurgitation.

Conclusions

In summary, establishing a specialized Marfan clinic appears to be an absolute necessity in order to closely monitor patients at risk and thus detect ominous changes along any segment of the aorta and other cardiac structures both before initial surgery and during the follow-up period.

References

1. Beighton P, de Paepe A, Danks D, Finidori G, Gedde-Dahl T, Goodman R, Hall JG, Hollister DW, Horton W, McKusick VA, Opitz JM, Pope FM, Pyeritz RE, Rimoin DL, Sillence D, Spranger JW, Thompson E, Tsipouras P, Viljoen D, Winship I, Young I (1988) International nosology of heritable disorders of connective tissue, Berlin, 1986. Am J Med Genet 29: 518–594
2. Bentall M, DeBono A (1968) A technique for complete replacement of ascending aorta Thorax 23: 338–339
3. Borst HG (1993) Composite aortic valve replacement and graft replacement of the ascending aorta plus coronary ostial reimplantation: How I do it. Semin Thorac Cardiovasc Surg 5: 71–73
4. Brown OR, DeMots H, Kloster FE (1975) Aortic root dilatation and mitral valve prolapse in Marfan's syndrome: An echocardiographic study. Circulation 52: 651–557
5. Burr HB, Krayenbuhl C, Sutton MSJ, Paneth M (1977) The mitral plication suture. J Thorac Cardiovasc Surg 73: 589
6. Cameron DE, Gott VL (1993) Composite aortic valve replacement and graft replacement of the ascending aorta plus coronary ostial reimplantation: How I do it. Semin Thorac Cardiovasc Surg 5: 63–65
7. Cabrol C, Pavie A, Gandjbakhch, Villemot JP, Guiraudon G, Laughlin L, Etievent Ph, Cham B (1981) Complete replacement of the ascending aorta with reimplantation of the coronary arteries: New surgical approach. J Thorac Cardiovasc Surg 81 (2): 309–315, 1981 Feb
8. Coselli JS, Crawford ES (1993) Composite aortic valve replacement and graft replacement of the ascending aorta plus coronary ostial reimplantation: How I do it. Semin Thorac Cardiovasc Surg 5: 55–62
9. David TE (1993) When, why, and how should the native aortic valve be preserved in patients with annuloaortic ectasia or Marfan syndrome? Semin Thorac Cardiovasc Surg 5: 93–96
10. Ennker J, Schubert C, Schneider R, Felix R, Hetzer R (1989) Postoperative Erfolgs- und Verlaufskontrollen thorakaler Aortenerkrankungen mittels Kernspintomographie. Langenbecks Arch Chir 374: 349–357
11. Ergin MA, Griepp RB (1993) When, why, and how should the native aortic valve be preserved in patients with annuloaortic ectasia or Marfan syndrome? Semin Thorac Cardiovasc Surg 5: 91–92
12. Gerbode F, Kerth WJ, Osborn JJ, Seker A (1962) Correction of mitral insufficiency by open operation. Ann Surg 155: 846

13. Gillinov AM, Hulyalkov A, Cameron DE, Cho PW, Greene PS, Reitz BA, Pyeritz RE, Gott VL (1994) Mitral valve operation in patients with the Marfan syndrome 107 (3): 724–731
14. Glesby MJ, Pyeritz RE (1989) Association of mitral valve prolapse and systemic abnormalities of connective tissue: A phenotypic continuum. JAMA 262: 523–528
15. Gott VL, Pyeritz RE, Cameron DE (1991) Composite graft repair of Marfan aneurysm of the ascending aorta: Results in 100 patients. Ann Thorac Surg 52: 38–45
16. Kouchoukos N (1993) Composite aortic valve replacement and graft replacement of the ascending aorta plus coronary ostial reimplantation: How I do it. Semin Thorac Cardiovasc Surg 5: 66–70
17. McKusick VA (1955) The cardiovascular aspects of Marfan's syndrome: A heritable disorder of connective tissue. Circulation 11: 321–342
18. Miller DC, Mitchell RS (1993) Composite aortic valve replacement and graft replacement of the ascending aorta plus coronary ostial reimplantation: How I do it Semin Thorac Cardiovasc Surg 5: 74–83
19. Miller DC (1993) The continuing dilemma concerning medical versus surgical management of patients with acute type B dissections. Sem Thorac Cardiovasc Surg 5 (1): 33–46
20. Morse RP, Rockenmacher S, Pyeritz RE, et al. (1990) Diagnosis and management of infantile Marfan. Pediatrics 86 (6): 888–895
21. Murdoch JL, Walker BA, Halpern BL, et al. (1972) Life expectancy and cause of death in the Marfan syndrome. N Engl J Med 286 (15): 804–808
22. Pyeritz RE (1993) The Marfan syndrome in Connective Tissue and its Heritable Disorders eds. Royce Steinmann, New York 1992, pp. 437–468, Wiley Liss Inc
23. Pyeritz RE (1991) Predictors of dissection of the ascending aorta in Marfan syndrome. Circulation 84: 351
24. Pyeritz RE, McKusick VA (1979) The Marfan syndrome: Diagnosis and management. N Engl J Med 300: 772–777
25. Tsipouras P, DelMastro R, Sarfarazi M, et al. (1992) Genetic linkage of the Marfan syndrome, ectopia lentis, and congenital contractural arachnodactyly to the fibrillin genes on chromosomes 15 and 5. The international Marfan syndrome collaborative study. N Engl J Med 326: 905–909
26. Sarsam M, Yacoub M (1993) Remodeling of the aortic valve anulus. J Thorac Cardiovasc Surg 105 (3): 435–438
27. Svensson LG, Crawford ES, Coselli JS, et al. (1989, suppl 1) Impact of cardiovascular operation on survival in the Marfan patient. Circulation 80 (3Pt1): I233–242
28. Zahka KG, Hensley C, Glesby M, et al. (1989, suppl) The impact of medical and surgical therapy on the cardiovascular prognosis of the Marfan syndrome in early childhood. J Am Coll Cardiol 13(2): 119A, 1989 Feb.

Authors' address:

Prof. Dr. med. R. Hetzer
German Heart Institute Berlin
Department of Cardiothoracic and Vascular Surgery
Augustenburger Platz 1
13353 Berlin
FRG

Marfan syndrome and pregnancy complicated by an acute dissecting aortic aneurysm DeBakey type I – A case report

A. von Hehn, R. Loose*, A. Bernhard*, I. Kötter-Thomsen**, R. Simon

University of Kiel, Departments of Cardiology, *Cardiovascular Surgery and **Gynaecology and Obstetrics, Kiel, FRG

We report the case of a 26-year-old woman who was in the 38th week of pregnancy (prima gravida); anamnestic intervention revealed that her mother had died at the age of 42 years because of a ruptured abdominal aortic aneurysm due to Marfan syndrome. During a routine CTG in the department for gynaecology and obstetrics, she complained of severe thoracic pain persisting since more than 24 h and independent from breathing, position and exercise, and was therefore transferred to our cardiology department for further investigation. She was 2.06 m in height and had a typical Marfan-habit (pes planus, thoracic lordosis, pectus deformity, joint hypermobility, arachnodactyly) (Fig. 1). Nevertheless, the diagnosis of Marfan syndrome had not been made previously. –

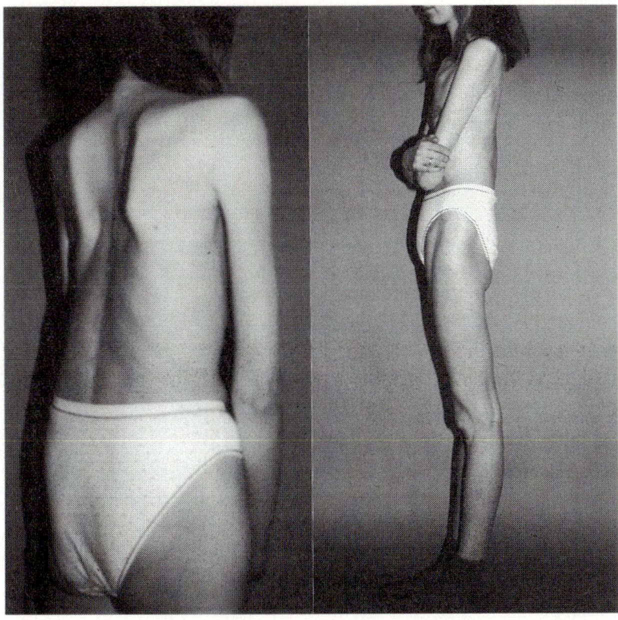

Fig. 1 Typical Marfan habit of our patient with 2.06 m height.

The ECG recordings were normal as well as the blood pressure; auscultation led to the preliminary diagnosis of severe aortic regurgitation and mitral insufficiency. The echocardiogram showed a huge dilatation of the bulbus aortae (6–7 cm) and with Doppler- and color-coded Doppler-echocardiography a severe aortic insufficiency and in addition a mitral regurgitation caused by a prolapse. The left ventricle was only slightly enlarged with unimpaired function. No signs of dissection could

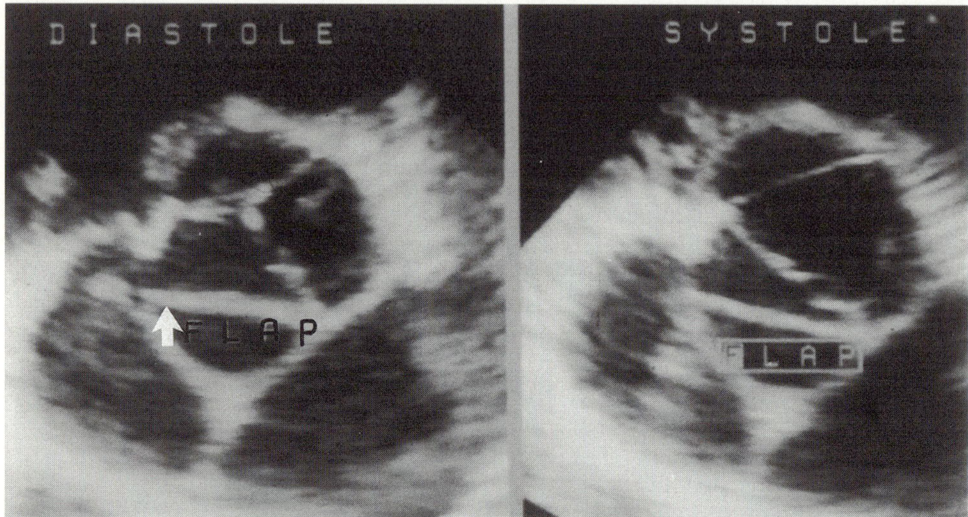

Fig. 2 Transesophageal echocardiography (TEE) at the level of the aortic valve: left atrium at the top, systolic phase on the right. Especially in diastole the horizontal intimal flap can clearly be differentiated below the "Mercedes-star".

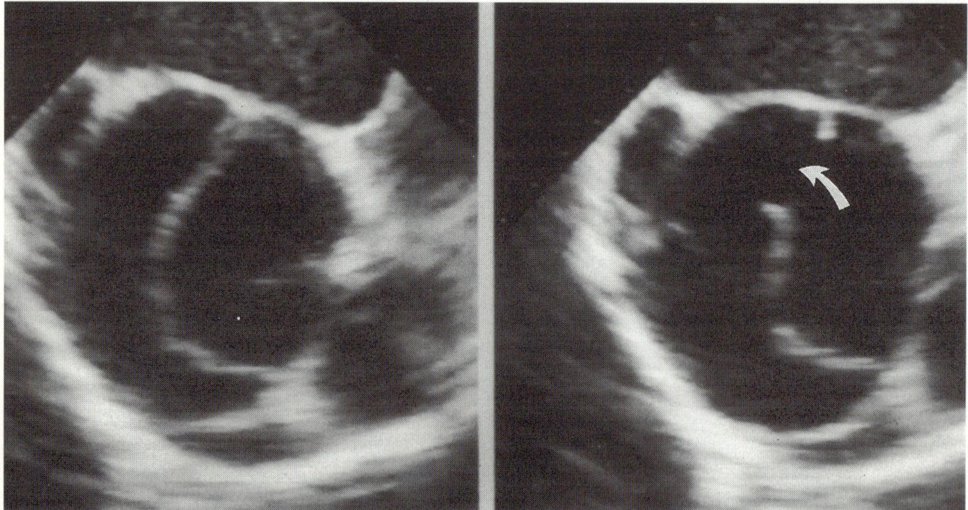

Fig. 3 TEE, same orientation, but left 1 cm above (i.e., cranial) the aortic cusps and right 1.5 cm further, with clear visualization of the large entry tear. The arrow demonstrates the flow direction from the (smaller) true lumen to the false lumen.

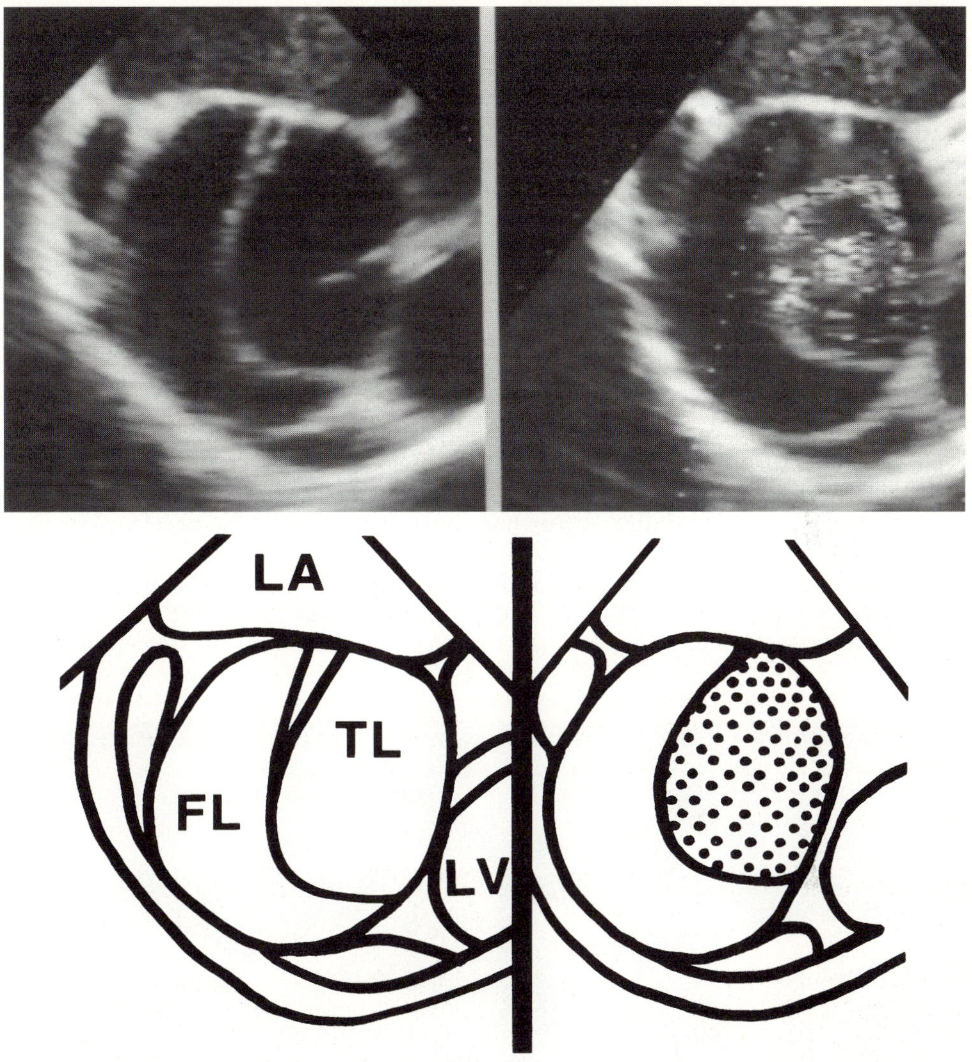

Fig. 4 TEE, same orientation. Color coded Doppler echocardiography on the right panel demonstrating antegrade flow in the true lumen (dotted on the graph) and no significant flow in the false lumen. Graph: LA = left atrium, FL = false lumen, TL = true lumen, LV = left ventricle.

be verified. The subsequent transesophageal approach (TEE) visualized directly above the level of the aortic cusps an additional structure, especially in the diastole clearly differentiated to be from the three cusps (Fig. 2) and suspicious for an intimal flap. Gradual pull-back of the transducer led to the detection of an entry in the intimal flap 1.5 cm above the cusps (Fig. 3) with color-coded Doppler-echocardiography differentiating between true and false lumen (Fig. 4). The intimal flap could he seen in the entire – visible part – of the ascending (diameter up to 6.5 cm), transverse (3.3 cm) – reaching into the truncus brachiocephalicus – and even in the descending part, but it could not be verified if the perfusion of the truncus was provided by the true or the false lumen. The diagnosis of an acute dissecting aortic aneurysm type I (DeBakey's classification) combined with a severe aortic regurgitation was confirmed. Further care of the patient in this emergency situation had to consider not only the risk of rupture of the aorta, acute heart failure and lethal complications, but also the pregnancy itself and the risk to the fetus. Thus, cardiologists, cardiovascular surgeons and obstetricians decided to immediately start the delivery with a sectio caesare in the cardiovascular operating room and to plan an aortic repair (valve replacement and aortic graft) within a one-time intervention. The delivery of a healthy female newborn (52 cm, 2880 g weight) was followed by the thoracotomy which presented a huge aorta with a dilatation starting directly at the bulbus aorta necessitating the implantation of a conduit-graft (33 mm diameter, 27 mm St.-Jude-Medical-prosthesis) and reimplantation of the coronary arteries. Because of a suture dehiscence a rethoracotomy became mandatory on the second post-operative day.

The newborn had no problems after delivery, but she also showed typical phenotypic signs of Marfan syndrome with echocardiographic proven slight enlargement of the ascending aorta, thus she was treated prophylactically with β-blockade (propanolol 2 mg/kg weight/daily); in further controls a drop of the acceleration time was verified.

The first echocardiographic control of our patient were normal with good position of the composite-graft (Fig. 5) and persistent dissection in the distal part of the ascending aorta – reaching into the truncus – the arch and the descending part

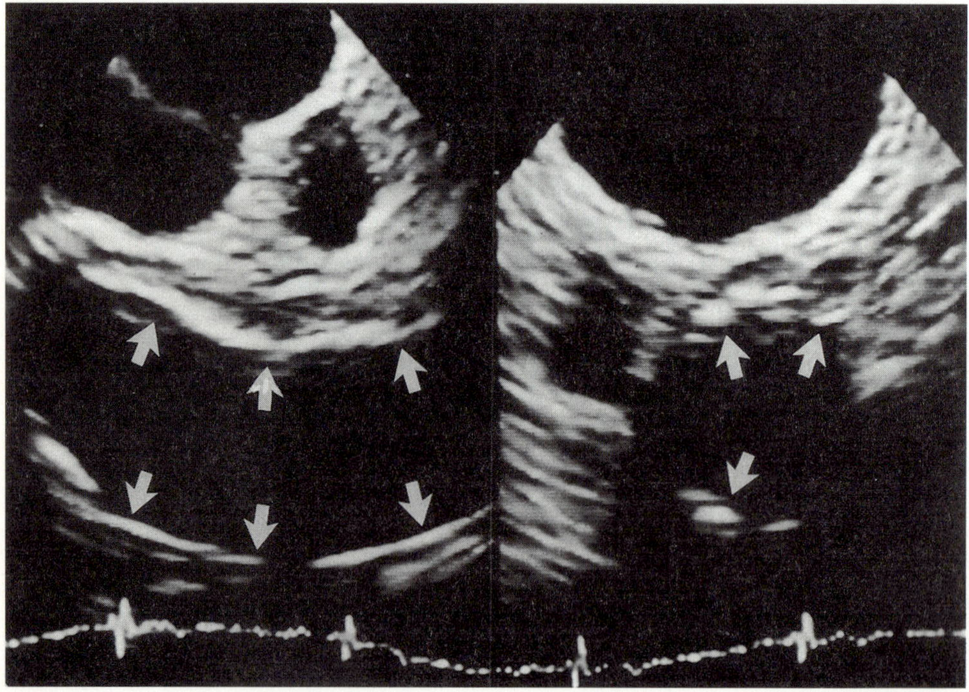

Fig. 5 TEE of the ascending aorta with the composite-graft (arrows) in the longitudinal plane left and horizontal plane on the right.

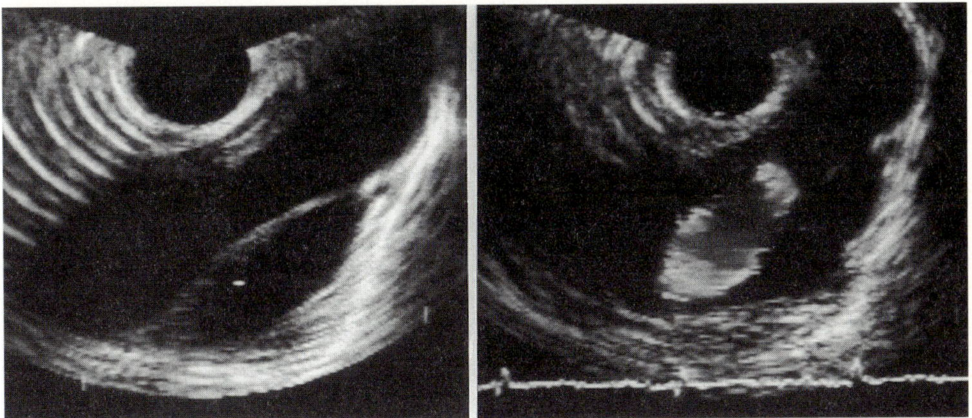

Fig. 6 TEE of the aortic arch with pesistent intimal flap and color coded Doppler on the right demonstrating antegrade flow in the true lumen (cranial) with no further entries or reentries and no significant flow in the false lumen (lower).

(Fig. 6); but in further controls we could document increasing diameter: in the second post-op year, the descending aorta reached 5.3 cm diameter, proven by CT scans and catheterization (showing normal anatomy of the coronary arteries and that the perfusion of the truncus was provided by the true lumen). We performed a close follow-up (6 months) with both transthoracic and TEE. After a subarachnoidal haemorrhage of unknown aetiology the medication was changed from cumarin to aspirin with a β-blocking agent leading to positive results in blood-pressure monitoring.

Discussion

This case report represents a wide panorama of typical problems in patients with Marfan syndrome which can be deleterious. The first point is the high percentage of patients in whom the diagnosis has not been confirmed before and done so only in emergency situations or by chance (1). In this case, it is astonishing because of the family history and the typical phenotype, and the height of 2.06 m in a female patient should have prompted further investigation. The second point is the problem of pregnancy in a Marfan patient itself, with a lethal risk of more than 50%, which had led to various recommendations (from total avoidance of pregnancy up to a calculated risk related to the aortic diameter (depending if < 4 cm or > 4 cm) and even more the problems in those patients in whom the diagnosis is first made during pregnancy. A literature review of the last 30 years revealed only four case reports of similar emergency situations at the end of pregnancy; the last (6) reported a lethal result in a patient presenting with a TIA and undiagnosed dissected aortic aneurysm (proven by the pathologist). But the special situation of our patient with a one-time obstetric-cardiovascular operation and delivery in the cardiovascular operating theatre (5) is unique. Furthermore, this report underlines the special impact of TEE in the diagnosis of aortic dissections because of its high sensitivity and specificity, thus being also an ideal method for planning the therapeutical management – answering almost all of the surgeons preoperative questions with mostly no need of other imaging techniques – as well as for the follow-up (3). There are also first reports about three-dimensional echocardiography (especially of the descending aorta) that perhaps allow better timing of a re-operation (4). Because of the time-course in our case there was no alternative for the immediate operation, the anatomical site allowing only implantation of a composite-graft (2) and in this emergency situation only a repair of the ascending part, because all complications are strongly related to the operation duration. There was no alternative to delivery by sectio caesare at the end of the 38th week; all was done without any significant problems. Only the time-point for re-operation for the mother is controversial, but most authors recommend it for a diameter exceeding 6 mm (1) or an increase of about 1 cm/year. Another reason for a second operation could be an increase of mitral regurgitation (4) caused by the prolapse (typically predominantly of the posterior leaflet).

References

1. de Belder MA, Child AH, Pumphrey CW (1989) Comment: The timing of aortic root replacement in Marfan's syndrome. Current Medical Literature: Cardiov. Med 8: 67–70
2. Gott VL, Pyeritz RE, Magovern GJ, Cameron DE, McKusick VA (1986) Surgical treatment of aneurysms of the ascending aorta in the Marfan syndrome. J Thorac Cardiovasc Surg 107: 724–731
3. von Hehn A, Nellessen U, Loose R, Simon R (1992) Follow-up of thoracic aortic aneurysms with biplane transesophageal echocardiography. Eur Heart J 13 (Abstr suppl): 131
4. von Hehn A (1994) First experience with the echocardiographic 3-D reconstruction of the thoracic aorta. Bildgebung/Imaging 61: 110–115
5. Kötter-Thomsen I, Weisner D, Lehmann-Willenbrock E, Swalve S, von Hehn A (1991) Marfan-Syndrom und Schwangerschaft, kompliziert durch das Aneurysma dissecans. Geburtsh Frauenheilk 51: 653–654
6. Menger H, Bedrossian-Pfingsten J (1991) Dissezierendes Aortenaneurysma in der Schwangerschaft mit neurologischer Symptomatik. Herz + Gefäße 11: 524–531

Authors' address:

Arist von Hehn, M.D.
Christian-Albrechts-Universität
I. Medizin-Klinik für Kardiologie
Schittenhelmstraße 12
FRG 24105 Kiel

Afternoon panel session

Moderated by Christian Cabrol and Roland Hetzer

HETZER: I think one of the very important questions, which is also important for our medical colleagues, is when would we consider operating on the ascending aorta, at which diameter and at what age, and whether there should be aortic valve incompetence or not. What do you think the criteria should be to suggest surgery for a patient?

HEINEMANN: In Hannover we would operate on any patient with an ascending aorta greater than 5 cm in diameter, below this only if the ascending aorta is distending rapidly, about half a centimeter per year, under close follow-up. For children it is very difficult. Dr. Albert from Memphis, Tennessee, has tried to calculate normograms for what is considered to be a normal aortic root in childhood which correlates diameter to body surface area. We have heard earlier on that this might not be very reliable.

COSELLI: We too have used about a 5-cm cut-off, with or without the presence of aortic valve insufficiency. If you are in a situation where you can provide a relatively safe operation with a very good early survival rate, you can be aggressive and offer these patients an operation at a relatively early stage.

BENTALL: I have had one tall Marfan patient rupture his aorta. He had only a 5-cm aortic root, and he fell off a haystack. In other words, it is possible for people to rupture their aortas in this disease, even when they are only 5 cm in a big man, the surface really does not enter into it. If Magdi is right, and I suspect he may be, that it is possible in increasing numbers to preserve the native valve successfully, then, one should perhaps even go down below that, down to about 4.5 cm, so that you have got a really beautiful non-dilated valve ring.

HETZER: This is a very good standpoint. As you have seen, we have also operated on some younger patients who had family members who had ruptured or dissected aortas at the age of 16 or 17 where obviously there was concern in the family. We operated on aortas of 4 or 4.5 cm diameter.

Sir YACOUB: For the patients with an aneurysm, with or without aortic regurgitation, we feel very strongly that if you are going to replace the valve then probably you should defer the operation because valve replacement is not advisable. But if you are going to repair the valve, then we take an aggressive attitude. We repair these valves – in teenagers – of 35 mm or more diameter, or 5 cm in adults, but more recently, in anybody with a dilated aortic sinus where it is definitely an aneurysm, before the valve becomes too incompetent. One important point which has been mentioned is that family history is a very important prognostic indicator, and therefore, in those with family history of dissection, we would be very aggressive about replacing.

ROBISCEK: 4.5 sounds like a good number to me. I would also operate on patients who had more than 50% of the diameter of the aorta distally. I would move towards surgery if the patient exhibits Marfan types. I operated on a patient who was 16 years old because his brother ruptured his aorta when he was 17. When the patient shows any signs of aortic regurgitation, I regard this as movement of the aortic root. It is unstable and I would proceed in that case with surgery. It might sound quite radical, but if you consider that in bona-fide Marfan's 90% of the patients die from complications of ascending aorta problem, maybe we should operate before dilatation occurs or whenever the slightest dilatation occurs. Concerning the term of annulo-aortic ectasia, it has generated considerable controversy. I would propose that we change it to aorto-annular ectasia because the annular ectasia never preceedes the aortic ectasia. It can be seen as an extension of the ascending aortic process into the annulus.

CABROL: First I take into account the evolution of the aneurysms. If it is between 5 or 6 cm in diameter I can follow closely whether it is increasing in size. If it does, of course, the indication is mandatory, otherwise it is debatable. Regarding the association with aortic insufficiency there also is an argument to operate on these patients. It is interesting what Magdi said, that it is important to operate these patients before aortic insufficiency has developed. If you do a good and appropriate cure of the ascending aorta, you may avoid the aortic insufficiency.

REIDEMEISTER: Is there any influence of the genetic screening in indication formation? Perhaps it is another policy in Marfan Syndrome compared to these "marfanoid" patients?

HETZER: This is a very important question. Here in Berlin we have also begun setting up a laboratory to do the fibrillin-producing fibroblast cultures as has been shown this morning. It might be very valuable to specify those patients who belong to the real Marfan group and those who we call "marfanoid," who have the aortic features of a Marfan patient, maybe some other slight features, but do not fulfill the required diagnostic criteria of Marfan syndrome.

Sir YACOUB: We were really fascinated this morning with the molecular approaches, and particularly, in trying to look at the relationship between genotype and phenotype and how that is going to show us some prognostic indicators. I am sure in the future we will have to look at that, but we are not there yet.

HEINEMANN: A small thing that we can do as surgeons is that if somebody comes in with an acute dissection, survives the operation, we should obtain quite a good family history in order to pick up families that are not aware of having some kind of connective tissue disease or Marfan syndrome.

INBERG: It is very important when you operate a patient with the so-called annulo-aortic ectasia to examine very carefully all the first-degree relatives. We echoed 500 first-degree relatives and many of those relatives without Marfan syndrome have dilatation of the aortic arch. Because of this follow-up, we have already operated patients without other symptoms in 5 cases. We are continuing with this follow-up. I think it is very important because I think the so-called annulo-aortic ectasia does not differ very much from the Marfan syndrome in this respect.

CABROL: We as cardiovascular surgeons must know that those patients have other problems and we must take advice from orthopedists and ophthalmologists. These patients must be very well checked and treated for all their problems.

COSELLI: I think that we as surgeons, in particular, in recommending rather aggressive therapy on patients in the very early phases of the disease, need to be very careful when we evaluate our own material to make sure that we are looking only at patients that do indeed have Marfan syndrome and that we are relatively certain of this and not "mixing apples and oranges" with our own data. In our own work, virtually every one of the patients in which we put in composite valve grafts for Marfan syndrome have aortic valve insufficiency. None of the aortic tissue which we removed is normal in pathological evaluation and 100% of the aortic valve leaflets have severe myxomatous degeneration as a minimum. If we are going to take our results out to long-term evaluations and recommend certain forms of therapy in patients in the early phases, we need to be certain that what we started with at the beginning is a comparable situation.

Sir YACOUB: I must object to the use of the term myxomatous degeneration of the aortic valve. We, too, made this mistake 20 years ago when we talked about floppy mitral and floppy aortic valve and myxomatous degeneration of the mitral and myxomatous degeneration of the aortic valve. When we looked afterwards, myxomatous degeneration occurs only in the mitral valve. If you look at the histology of the aortic valve in Marfan or non-Marfan with aortic regurgitation, there is no myxomatous degeneration. This term sometimes is used too easily.

NIENHABER (Hamburg): What role does the angiogram still play in the diagnosis, and do you need that for the definitive diagnosis of dissection?

HETZER: I must apologize for the structure of this meeting today that we have somewhat neglected the diagnostic and cardiology part. I am very well aware of this, but being a surgeon, of course, I put greater emphasis on the questions that we had about it. I believe modern echocardiography replaces angiography in most of the cases. In all patients under the age of 40 or 50 years, we would not ask for an angiogram in elective patients, and of course not in acute dissection.

INBERG: In Turku we always use angiography for postoperative monitoring to see what happens at the coronary orifices. We have seen some dilatation in our group of 92 patients, but we do not know the clinical significance of this dilatation.

NIENHABER: Does that mean that you even need a coronary angiogram?

HETZER: May I ask my echocardiographer to respond to this. I am in the lucky position to have an echocardiographer who tells me where the coronary ostia are in those patients.

SINIAWSKI (Berlin): We can demonstrate coronary ostia in Marfan syndrome in nearly 100% of the cases and we are measuring mainstem flow velocities in the left mainstem. We look at the morphology and see how it develops over time.

HETZER: I would like to ask the other surgeons on the panel what kind of diagnostics they need in acute and in elective cases.

HEINEMANN: We have come to the conclusion that in the acute type-A dissections we do not have time for angiography, sometimes also not for CT scans, so if we have an echo that we can thereby recognize the dissection, and if it fits with the symptoms the patient is presenting with, that is sufficient. Everybody who goes into the OR to undergo surgery for suspected acute type A dissection gets a transesophageal probe during induction of the anesthesia. For the elective patients, we have been very comfortable with the new technique of a spiral CT with the ability of 3-D reconstruction. We do perform angiographies if there is a suspicion of a malperfusion of a vital abdominal or other aortic branches, and we do perform coronary angiography in all the risk groups especially in all the elderly patients with chronic type A and especially chronic type B dissections because these patients usually have a long-standing history of hypertension and may have all the risk factors for coronary artery disease.

COSELLI: Our approach is quite similar. We take patients based on echocardiography, particularly in an emergency situation, directly to the operating room. We use intraoperative transesophageal echocardiography in every case. It is also particularly helpful in any type of valve repair procedure. In patients with distal aortic disease, we still like to use aortography to demonstrate the patency and location and the relationship of the branch vessels, the relationship to the true and the false lumen to re-attach these vessels.

BENTALL: The only thing I would like to add is that the MRI scan can be extremely helpful in dissection. We were lucky in having one with us at Hammersmith for 12 years. I would recommend it if you have one. You can certainly see coronaries by using that.

Sir YACOUB: I would like to make two points, one is that I entirely agree that there is no indication for angiography except for defining peripheral coronary arterial disease. For postoperative control the MRI imaging with a fair technique would clearly show the proximal coronary arteries now for 4 or 5 cm beyond the orifices, and furthermore, it will give you flow velocity and tell you whether there is dilatation and whether there is a hemodynamic problem.

ROBISCEK: We usually do an angiographic work-up before we take the history and physical on most of our patients. In emergency situations we use our CT scan quite extensively, and lately, we are experimenting with intravascular ultrasound in dissections which appears to be very promising. I would say that in about 80% of the cases we do angiograms, and "horrible addicts" do CT scans as well.

CABROL: Yes, we like to have an angiography of the coronary arteries, when it is not an emergency case, in order to know precisely what to do, but in an emergency I think that transesophageal echocardiography is a very useful tool and allows us to do good work.

CHILD: I would like to ask whether any of you have had successful pregnancies in women with Marfan syndrome after aortic root replacement and how you would manage them. I have 2 women who have had successful pregnancies, but there is always the question of whether to use anticoagulant or not, antibiotics, and do you do Cesarean section?

HETZER: I am not aware if any of our female patients whom we have operated has had a pregnancy, but we have taken this into consideration. This is also one of the reasons why we try to preserve the valve; it started as a valve-preservation technique, particularly in young women. We also have some patients who are not on coumadin, even with polycarbon mechanical valves, but just on aspirin. Of course aspirin is not a good solution for pregnancy either, but it may be easier to handle.

HEINEMANN: We are also trying to pursue techniques to preserve the native aortic valve. The other option that we should not forget is the homograft valve for an elective root replacement in a young woman so we do not have to have any anticoagulation. There is only one patient whom I can remember with the Marfan syndrome where we encountered pregnancy, but this was a dissection which occurred during pregnancy. This was during the eighth month, so she got her composite graft and the baby at the same time. We did the Cesarean section first under emergency conditions and then replaced the ascending aorta.

Sir YACOUB: We have experience with one patient who had four successful pregnancies, two Marfan and two non-Marfan detected children, having had a homograft before. Equally, we had one patient, a young female doctor who presented in her sixth month of pregnancy with an acute dissection. We preserved her valve and tried to preserve the baby unsuccessfully. We lost the baby on the sixth day postoperatively. I understand she is pregnant again.

PYERITZ: Two of our patients' post-composite grafts have become pregnant: in one, the pregnancy was not successful for spontaneous termination reasons, another patient successfully carried a pregnancy, but this was a patient who had a type A dissection. She extended the dissection during delivery and wound up having repair shortly thereafter. We have just reviewed the series of patients who electively undertook pregnancy before composite graft surgery, these were women who were advised that their risk was increased for dissection or some other untoward cardiovascular event, but whose aortic roots were 40 mm or less at the time they undertook the pregnancy. We have 20 women who have had over 30 pregnancies. There is no increased risk to the fetus. There is no increased risk of obstetrical complications and, with two exceptions, the women showed no particular dilatation of their aortic root during the pregnancy. They had echocardiography every 6 to 8 weeks beginning before conception on through 6 months after delivery. There were two women: one with a 46-mm root and moderate aortic regurgitation who suffered a type A dissection during pregnancy, and one woman who showed a very rapid increase in her aortic root from 46 to 70 mm during pregnancy. She had elective repair shortly after delivery. So I think that the outlook for a woman whose root is not greatly enlarged, 40 mm or less, is not equal to the population average certainly, but it is not terrible. So these women can probably undergo elective pregnancy before they have an aortic root repair.

CHILD: We had one young lady who dissected at 4.2 cm. Her father also dissected at 4.2 cm. So I think the family history needs to be taken into account when counseling young women about pregnancy.

HETZER: Coming back to the homograft, you have not experienced any dilatation of a homograft in a Marfan patient?

Sir YACOUB: No. I mean, you can have degeneration but the homograft tissue would continue to be from the donor and I do not think that the fibrillin gene will affect the homograft as such.

We had one patient where the homograft root had leaked about 3 months after the operation. This person, 6 years after surgery, has mild to moderate regurgitation and he will require replacement. I have always maintained that the annulus in Marfan, as I have said, is normal and I always try very hard to use what I call a homo-vital valve, which happens to be very small. The mistake was I put a small aortic root, smaller than what should have been used, it was 2.1 in a root which was 2.5. If you have a homograft which is 2.5, it should be sufficient for a patient with Marfan if you replace the root. It does not get stretched out. If you get too ambitious and put too small a homograft, it will be stretched.

HETZER: I fully agree that the dilatation of the annulus, as you say, may not be due to Marfan syndrome. But in some of those Marfan patients, you are confronted with huge annulae, sometimes a 31 valve is probably just good enough to put in there. I have always been against using homografts in Marfan patients because the annulus might tear apart or it may be too big for the homograft.

Sir YACOUB: The annulus itself is not very large. You get this appearance of a huge root because of the spread out of the aneurysm. But when you use a homograft of about 2.5, it sits very well as a root replacement. At one stage, we used to plicate the root, now we do not even plicate the root because you put it right down on the fibrous annulus.

CABROL: I also think the annulus is less dilated than it appears. It is the enlargement of the sinuses of valsalva which give this appearance more than the real, actual diameter of the annulus.

CARLOS MESTRES (Barcelona): I presume that most of you on the panel use mechanical composite valves, with the exception of Prof. Yacoub. I have quite a few questions. The first is, provided you want to use biological tissue to repair the valve, what is the best? You mentioned that the trend is now toward valve repair if possible, but on the other hand, we have to be reminded that a potential disadvantage is that you definitely may leave bad tissue in the form of valve leaflets themselves, and secondly, the risk of late infective endocarditis seems to be a little higher with valve repair. I would like to know a bit more about your experience with homografts. How large, on average, was the size of the homografts you implanted in Marfan patients and how large was the diameter of the homograft which failed late, and also the technique you use for aortic valve replacement in Marfan patients. Free hand plus Dacron tube, root inclusion technique, or full aortic root replacement?

Sir YACOUB: Why one perceives that the aortic valve is abnormal; we still think that being your own valve and lacking even the myxomatous degeneration, like what happens in the mitral valve, it is the best choice to preserve it. When we started repairing the myxomatous valves everybody was saying you are repairing very abnormal tissue, it is going to leak, it is much better to do a replacement. Now, very few people will disagree that the repair of even myxomatous valves in the mitral position lasts. In the aortic position, histologically even, there is not as bad a degeneration as in the mitral position. So, we are hopeful that that will hold. We feel that the ones which failed actually failed early, and technically they were not very good or we extended the cusps and, therefore, valve repair currently is still, to my way of thinking, better than any other valve, better even than homografts. The homo-vital homografts are performing very well, but I do not think as well as one's own tissue. The size of the homografts, as I mentioned, averaged 2.4 to 2.6. I have used composite grafts in all the patients except one in the early series where I plicated the existing root and then put a free hand.

HETZER: I would like to raise another field in the discussion and that is the mitral valve in Marfan patients. Quite a number of the real Marfan patients develop huge mitral annuli and mitral incompetence and in some we had to go back years after ascending replacement and also replace the mitral valve. Each time when I operated such an aortic valve or aortic aneurysm, I looked down into the left ventricle and I saw a big mitral valve, even if it was competent at the time of the operation; I often asked myself whether it would be worthwhile to do at least some mitral annulus shortening in order to prevent later mitral dilatation. We have a study underway examining all of those patients and the prospect of later development of mitral incompetence. I would like to ask the opinions of the panel.

Sir YACOUB: I think that mitral regurgitation and aortic regurgitation is not a continuum. It is almost a different phenotype. I have seen people, young females, presenting with mitral regurgitation mainly in a family, although they are Marfan, with minimal or no aortic root dilatation. The opposite is true in patients with a large aorta and aortic regurgitation, although they have a floppy mitral valve, they tend to leak much less. We have not seen attrition and what happens later is that they get more distal aneurysms like we have seen with Dr. Coselli's series where they rupture or have aortic replacement, but surprisingly not late mitral regurgitation, even 20 years later.

HETZER: This was the original concern I brought up. I wonder what happened to those big mitral valves, and the echocardiographer tells me often that a patient, although he has a competent mitral valve, has a huge annulus, like maybe 8 cm diameter or more. I thought to myself, maybe in a few years I have to go back and operate on this.

Sir YACOUB: But we know from the natural history of floppy valves, for example, we have done a study like that published in Circulation in the 1970's, where patients had the murmur with a floppy valve, with a dilated myxomatous valve for 25 years before they started having significant mitral regurgitation. So, to step in before it happens, might be too aggressive.

COSELLI: In Dr. Crawford's 179 or so Marfan patients, only 2 at a later stage required reoperation specifically directed at mitral valvular insufficiency and those were at 7 and 11 years. One of the patients in the 66 operations that I showed who required re-do composite valve graft replacement also had severe mitral insufficiency and required a mitral valve replacement at the time. That is only 3 in well over 200 cases, so I am not sure that it would warrant enough to go ahead and do anything at the initial operation for these people who almost all have floppy mitral valves and some mitral prolapse.

PYERITZ: I think there is general agreement that the Marfan patient who comes to cardiac surgery with an aortic dissection has a poor long-term prognosis for avoiding surgery in the future. The issue that I think needs to be addressed is what about the patient who has an elective aortic composite graft or reconstruction of some sort who does not have a dissection. What is that patient's long-term prognosis for developing distal aortic difficulties, aneurysms in other vessels, and so forth? I have a bias. I think the long-term perspective is very good. On the other hand, I keep all of such patients on β-blockade for the rest of their lives, or at least until something better comes along. I would like to hear your perspectives.

Sir YACOUB: I thought that you would be the person who would be able to answer that question for us because you are the only person who has a prospective randomized trial which you said you would be publishing in the New England Journal of Medicine. We take the view that it is almost unethical not to put them on β-blockers. That is just by heresay and it makes sense that lowering the DP/DT and lowering the blood pressure must be a good thing. So we put all our patients on varying degrees of β-blockade. We do not know how effective that is, however, because we still see, and you have heard from almost everybody, that there is a late problem. ACE inhibition seems to lower coronary events because of the RAS System being expressed in the heart and it might be that the RAS has something to do with the aorta as well. So that is yet another molecular thing to pursue. The next question is, how effective is it in prevention, and then further, what are the different prognostic indicators? What makes one patient have a very rapid deterioration or rupture? You were trying to answer that for us in the morning showing what molecular changes and how there are several defects, point mutations or deletions or something, which can account for that. We are dealing with a heterogenous group of patients. Not one thing is going to prevent the problem, is it?

ROBISCEK: First of all, as far as I know, there is no proof in Marfan prospective studies that either blood-pressure-lowering medication or β-blockers are of any benefit. The habit of putting people on them is based on animal experiments. But all the animal experiments, in the turkey and the mice, are not done on a Marfan model, they are done on a hypertensive model. So I would even ask, is it ethical to put these patients on β-blockers.

PYERITZ: This morning I reported the 10-year follow-up of the randomized control trial of propranolol in Marfan patients that shows definite benefit both in a life table analysis and in the rate of dilatation of the aortic root. The issue remains, as to whether that is pertinent to the distal aorta. I would remind the audience that the aorta is not a homogeneous structure itself, that the amount of elastic tissue decreases as one moves distally, the amount of collagenous material increases as one moves distally. The hemodynamic forces acting on the aorta are different distally than they are proximally. Inserting some sort of rigid tube in the ascending aorta may well influence the characteristics distally over the long term. I think there is clear need here for a randomized trial. I think β-blockade is clearly indicated in patients before surgery, we can debate when to begin it, but after surgery I think there is room, not only for debate, but for a very good study. We have enough patients here that we could probably do a multicenter one.

HETZER: We have a number of patients without dissection who developed aneurysms at distal parts of the aorta. I agree that all of those patients should be kept on blood pressure-reducing agents at least. I think that the concept is probably debatable. We use β-blockade or ACE-inhibitors or both. Very close follow-up should be done. That is also one of the things I wanted to discuss, for instance, every half year comparable control studies under a comparable or similar method, that is what we usually do with such patients.

GERHARD ZUMSTEIN (President of the Swiss Marfan Foundation): Since I get the permission and chance to ask and raise the last easy question, by the way I would like to thank you gentlemen in the name of all Marfan organizations, those present and the others not present, and in the name of all Marfan-affected people because we are watching your work very closely and we will, of course, within our journals and newsletters, talk about this gathering, this important congress in Berlin. So thank you again very much. Here is my question. One of the tougher decisions to make is often when to operate on your child. Children needing operations are mostly severely affected, otherwise you would not talk about this at that young age. So my question is, has there been agreement on any suggestion that intervention should not take place before the aneurysm in the ascending aorta has reached double the diameter of the arch? Has there been any consent among you? If, why, or what other means do you have to judge when to intervene.

Sir YACOUB: I think I will have to agree with that because the criteria we have is 3.5 in a teenager, which would be the double diameter of the arch, and 5 in an adult, which again would be the double. So I think, yes there is some agreement. I speak for myself.

HETZER: The smallest aortic bulb that we have operated was 3.5 cm in a child. We conducted a valve-preserving procedure.

GERHARD ZUMSTEIN: So in an expressive case at the age of 12 and just below 4 cm, having grown 2 mm in the last 6 months, what do you think about this?

COSELLI: I think when it comes to making that decision, even in children as we mentioned earlier, a couple of other factors have to be thrown in. One of them I think you have already alluded to. One is a stable aortic size and another one is that you have a documented progression of a relatively brief period of time. I think we would all be more aggressive.

HETZER: It entails an operative risk of close to 0 to perform an operation at this stage, on the other hand, the concern of the parents is certainly valid, especially if there is a very strong family history. We also would rather operate on such a patient. I think we can now close the discussion. We probably could go on. Of course for an organizer it's very good to see that the interest is greater than the time available. I'd like to thank all the participants, the speakers, the great gentlemen who came here, and the specialists of the basic sciences, and also the discussants. I also thank the audience for its patience and I'm very grateful to my co-workers, Frau Fissenewert and Frau Dr. Gehle, who have done most of the work to organize this symposium, and again I thank the companies which made it possible to host this symposium. Thank you very much.